Attending Others

Attending Others

A Doctor's Education in Bodies and Words

Brian Volck

CASCADE *Books* · Eugene, Oregon

ATTENDING OTHERS
A Doctor's Education in Bodies and Words

Cascade Books
An Imprint of Wipf and Stock Publishers
199 W. 8th Ave., Suite 3
Eugene, OR 97401

www.wipfandstock.com

PAPERBACK ISBN: 978-1-62032-728-9
HARDCOVER ISBN: 978-1-4982-8877-4

Cataloguing-in-Publication data:

Volck, Brian.

   Attending others : a doctor's education in bodies and words / Brian Volck.

   xvi + 200 pp. ; 23 cm. Includes bibliographical references.

   ISBN 978-1-62032-728-9 (paperback) | ISBN 978-1-4982-8877-4 (hardback)

   1. Volck, Brian. 2. Pediatricians—United States—Biography. I. Title.

RJ43.66 V58 2016

Manufactured in the U.S.A.   03/07/16

"Paying Attention" originally appeared in a different form as "In the Details," in *DoubleTake*, winter, 2002.

"Wendell and Me" originally appeared in a different form as "Mr. Berry Goes to Medical School: Notes toward Unspecializing a Healing Art," in Shuman, Joel James and L. Roger Owens, eds. *Wendell Berry and Religion: Heaven's Earthly Life*. Lexington, KY: University of Kentucky Press, 2009.

Excerpts from *Slow Pilgrim: The Collected Poems* by Scott Cairns, Copyright © 2015 by Scott Cairns. Used with permission www.paracletepress.com

Excerpt from "Those of Us Who Think We Know." Copyright © 1976 by Stephen Dunn, from *New and Selected Poems 1974-1994* by Stephen Dunn. Used by permission of W.W. Norton & Company, Inc.

Author's Note: The names of patients, their families, and some others have been changed and/or had significant details altered to protect anonymity.

To the children who taught me
and for Jill, who gives me
new ways to see, reasons to sing,
and time to write.

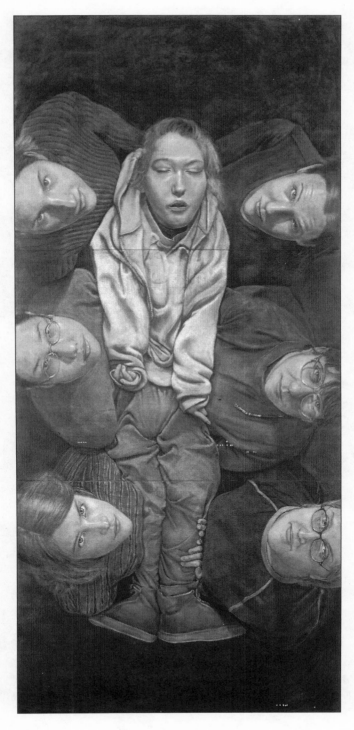

"Carry Me" by Tim Lowly

"I fear bodies, I tremble to meet them. What is this Titan that has possession of me? Talk of mysteries!"[1]

—Henry David Thoreau

"And the words we find
are always insufficient, like love,
though they are often lovely
and all we have."[2]

—Stephen Dunn

1. Thoreau, *The Maine Woods*, in *Henry David Thoreau*, 646.
2. Dunn, Stephen, "Those of Us Who Think We Know" in *New and Selected Poems 1974–1994*, 58.

Contents

Acknowledgments

No book is truly written alone. No author is an island, entire of itself. Many people helped make this memoir possible. My debt to them endures, and I can now do little more than mention several by name and offer my inadequate thanks.

First and foremost, I am forever indebted to the children I have cared for and the families who welcomed me into their lives, however briefly. The company of children is the reason I stayed in medicine when I might have done otherwise. Kids remain my best, most honest teachers. I hope some received nearly as much from me as they gave. Thanks in particular to the Navajo Nation and the people of Honduras for the honor of caring for your children.

My best professional mentors—attendings, nurse practitioners, nurses, and therapists—taught me by example (and sometimes in so many words) that our first task is to care for the child, no matter how difficult the circumstances. In the long run, nobody really cares how bad your night on call was. What matters is how your patients did. Among the institutions that shaped my medical practice and acquainted me with some of the finest healers alive are: Washington University in St. Louis School of Medicine, University Hospitals of Cleveland/Rainbow Babies and Children's Hospital, Tuba City Regional Health Care Center, Northern Kentucky Family Health, University Pediatrics and Internal Medicine, Cincinnati Children's Hospital Medical Center, the Indian Health Service, and Shoulder to Shoulder, Inc.

Thanks also to the students, residents, and fellows I've had the good fortune to teach and who taught me in return through perceptive questions, not all of which I may have appreciated at the time.

To the writer-mentors I name in the text: I hope I have done you justice. Special thanks to the Seattle Pacific University MFA in creative writing and the Generations in Dialogue program through the Institute for Advanced Catholic Studies at the University of Southern California. Several chapters began as essays in my MFA thesis and I owe a lasting debt to Leslie Leyland Fields and Robert Clark for their perceptive critiques and needed encouragement. Other chapters were born between gatherings with the 2013–2015 cohort of Mullin Fellows through the Institute. I treasure the lessons learned and friendships made at these two fine programs. The following writers read one or more chapters—some long before I knew there was a book there—and offered suggestions ranging from helpful to transformative: Lisa Ampleman, Randy Boyagoda, Robert Clark, Robert Coles, Leslie Leyland Fields, Diane Glancy, David Griffith, Paula Huston, Kelly Foster Lundquist, William Loizeaux, Samuel Martin, Richard Rodriguez, Jenny Shank, Joel Shuman; Kathleen Tarr, and Greg Wolfe.

Thank you to the people and places offering a quiet place to write and plan, including: Camp Casey, Whidbey Island; St. Johns College, Santa Fe; Sage Hill B&B, Navajo Nation; and the Monastery of Christ in the Desert, Abiquiu. Endless thanks to Greg Wolfe, the Glen Workshop, and all my friends associated with *Image*, for showing me how this work is done and continuing to encourage me when this memoir became "the damn memoir." I owe a special debt to the visual artists who helped me see bodies and persons more clearly, especially Tim Lowly, Barry Moser, and my brother, John Volck.

Thanks to the families, colleagues, and friends who reviewed portions of the book that refer to them and letting me know what I got wrong. The resulting truths are yours and any remaining errors entirely mine. An avalanche of gratitude goes to Diana Hu and Steve Holve: you are the doctors I want to be when I grow up. Thank you for your boundless hospitality whenever I come to the Navajo Nation.

Thanks to the patient folks at Cascade, especially Christian Amondson, Rodney Clapp, Jon Stock, and Matt Wimer. I hope the resulting manuscript was worth the wait.

Thanks to my children, Will, Peter, and Maria, raised in a not-normal family, including a father who could have made a lot more money sticking with doctoring and dropping this writing nonsense. Perhaps some of my weirdness will be clearer to you after reading this. By teaching me the

First Lesson of Parenthood often and well, you transformed my practice of pediatrics and writing.

And thanks beyond reckoning to Jill Huppert, my wife, my chief supporter, and my first and best reader. You made this book possible.

Chapter One

A Wedding

Navajo Nation,
Northern Arizona

THE DIRT ROAD RUNNING north from Route 264 soon turns rough, where the car rumbles and shudders over sinuous tire grooves and long, corrugated flats. Washboard roads jar less when taken at speed, but this evening we've joined a slow procession of pickup trucks and SUVs on our way to a Navajo wedding. The groom is on horseback at the head of the line, and no one is in a hurry. Kalene rides in the passenger seat of my car. Kalene is a Navajo friend I first met twenty years ago, when I was a doctor at the Indian hospital in Tuba City, on the western part of the Navajo Reservation. My sixteen year-old daughter, Maria, sits in back, talking to Kalene's cousin about horses, school, and life on the Rez.

The late June afternoon is pleasant, but we've shut the windows against the dust stirred up by the cars ahead. The sun lingers in the western sky as if reluctant to leave. Raking light skims sandstone blufftops. Scattered boulders and a lone, ramshackle house throw lengthening shadows eastward. Traditional Navajo weddings begin after sundown, and Kalene reassures me we'll arrive before dusk.

"We're getting close," she says. "Just a little past that bend." From experience, I know what's close to a Navajo may seem far to an Anglo like me, but there's no rushing things, and our pace gives me time to ponder. Why, for instance, should I be so fortunate as to be here, in such company and

1

in this car, on our way to a wedding? In the five years my wife, Jill, and I
lived and worked full time on the Navajo Reservation, we were invited to
one wedding, and only in our last year. The invitation came from one of
Jill's co-workers, and Jill went for the both of us. I had to work at the hospital that day and couldn't attend. Only later did I begin to understand what
I'd missed, how rarely Anglos are asked to such events, except by Navajo
who've come to know you well enough to consider you extended family. The
Navajo practice of *k´e*, usually—if inadequately—translated as "kinship," is
one of those things Anglos—or as the Navajo say, "*bilagáanas*"—aren't likely
to grasp. There's a reason the Navajo language—*Diné bizaad*—was used as
a military code by US Marines in the Pacific during World War II, and the
complex, nuanced culture it gives voice to is every bit as challenging for *bilagáanas* to learn. One grows to accept gifts of friendship and hospitality as
moments of grace, like rounding a bend in a desolate canyon and finding a
cactus in full bloom: yellow, blood red, or magenta petals stretching toward
the sun. And here we are, my daughter and I, on our way to a wedding.

The groom nudges his horse leftward onto a sandy lane, and the parade of vehicles follows him toward a traditional Navajo hogan. At lane's
end, cars park on flat patches of hard, red earth. I try to do the same, but
my wheels spin freely in a sand drift. Rocking the car forward and reverse,
forward and reverse, I shimmy out while wedding guests shout words of
advice. My daughter, born in Guatemala, can pass for Navajo with her long,
straight, black hair, and café au lait skin. I'm the lone white guy and the only
driver stuck in the sand. My attempts to blend in have failed.

I look for a better place to park, find an open stretch of dirt next to
a pickup truck, and pull in. I haven't brought the car to a full stop when
Kalene opens the passenger door, steps out, and says, as if to explain her
sudden hurry, "I'm going to find a seat in the hogan."

"We can go inside?" I say to myself. I hadn't known what to expect, but
I had imagined we'd stand at a distance and not see much of the ceremony.
We follow Kalene, all of us stepping from the car into evening air pungent
with pinyon smoke and grilling mutton. The hogan stands twenty yards
away: a traditional, eight-sided Navajo home with a sooty metal chimney
poking from the center of the roof and a single doorway facing, as always,
to the east. This hogan is spacious, well maintained, with sturdy walls and
double-paned windows. A neighboring building—a house the size and
shape of a doublewide trailer—stands to the north of the hogan with all the
lights on. I suspect that's the everyday home of the bride's family, while the
hogan is used sparingly, for special occasions.

We walk to the east face of the hogan and spy tables and chairs arranged under a tarp, sheltered from the unlikely event of rain. Several men

tend a grill nearby while others unload bags of food and heavy coolers from a pickup. A few stand empty-handed, talking in voices barely above a whisper. Maria and I follow Kalene to the hogan door, and she beckons us inside. We follow into the warm, well-lit interior, and I'm once again struck by the nonchalance with which Navajo extend their staggering hospitality. Kalene and Maria sit on the north side, to the right of the east-facing door, with the women. I join the men to the left, and scan the interior to get my bearings, noticing again that I'm the only *bilagáana*, while my daughter blends in like a local. North and south windows open to gathering darkness. Pinyon branches crackle in the iron belly of a wood stove near the room's center. What light remains flashes from the polished silver of turquoise necklaces and earrings as the guests, dressed in their Navajo finest, turn to one another, speaking in undertones. The groom sits on the dirt floor alongside his saddle on the west side of the hogan, talking to an impressive older man, whom I recognize as Kalene's father. He's doing what older men do at weddings: calming the nervous groom. The younger man feigns confidence and ease in his stiff white shirt, concho belt, silver necklace, and cloth headband. He shoots a glance toward the door whenever someone enters. For all the differences between this wedding and others I've attended, including my own, some things are clearly the same: the groom grows twitchy and the bride arrives when she chooses, but not one minute before.

"Hey, doc!" a voice calls from behind me. I turn to see Philip, Kalene's brother in law, sitting by the open south window. He gives me a thumbs-up, perhaps congratulating me on getting here in one piece, perhaps acknowledging that I haven't yet offended anyone with *bilagáana* behavior, perhaps just to say hello. He leans forward and says softly, "Make sure you sit up front, so you can see." Other family members gesture me forward, closer to the coming action. A woman kneels by the wood stove, opens the cast iron door, and lights a small stick, blowing on the lit end as it smolders. The dark red of her velveteen blouse shimmers in the firelight. Maria's across from me, talking quietly to Kalene.

We're waiting for the *hatal łii*—the traditional healer who will lead the ceremony—and the bride, who will arrive soon enough in a white blouse, skirt, and squash blossom necklace. For now, though, in this in-between time of waiting, I sit as if in a doorway between the little I know and the enormity I don't, pondering how fortunate I am to be welcomed here, in this place on earth and this event few *bilagáanas* ever see. Surely this isn't something I've earned. This is grace, and I'm learning, at long last, to receive it as a gift.

I have enough affection for my Navajo friends and their complex, changing culture, to know this: I'm not Indian. That's another gift I received

from these people and this place, a gift that encouraged me to discover who
I am from my own traditions, origins, and story. Emmanuel Levinas, a twentieth century philosopher, insisted that anyone who has yet to encounter
someone as Other—as truly and challengingly different as the Navajo are to
me—is like someone asleep. For Levinas, the encounter with the Other calls
the person into being. I admire Navajo culture without, I hope, idealizing it.
I know the tradition to be as messy, flawed, life-giving, and beautiful as my
own. It my encounter with that Other that called me into deeper engagement with my origins and traditions.

One reason I'm here is obvious, though. I'm a doctor. It was as a pediatrician that I met Kalene. It's as a doctor that Philip knows me. Not many
bilagáanas are invited to Navajo weddings, but the privilege of caring for
the bodily health of others opened the door. By virtue of what doctors know
and, perhaps more importantly, what they can do, we're granted special access to the bodies and lives of patients. It shocks me to hear what people
I've just met are willing to share, not because I'm a good listener, but simply
because I'm a doctor. Otherwise reticent persons reveal astonishing intima-
cies to their physician. I know many things about medicine, and am grateful
for the scientific training I received along the way, yet this other side of my
work remains a mysterious and surprising gift. It wasn't a significant part of
my formal curriculum. I acquired what little I know about this part of my
profession—some call it "art"—more by accident than design.

The Latin root of the English word, "education," means "to lead out."
My most important lessons in doctoring occurred after I left the teaching
hospital and entered what is tellingly called "practice." Practices come with
history and traditions, ways of doing things that are neither arbitrary nor
immutable. Enduring practices are adaptable, alive. They abide in women
and men who learned from mentors and teach those who follow, each generation working toward a shared end forever beyond human grasp. Practice
doesn't make perfect, though it can make better, wiser, and kinder. Physicians are always practicing.

* * * *

It's sometimes revealing to view one practice from another. I love deserts and
love to raft the rivers that flow through them. When river rafters scout a major rapid in the Grand Canyon, pausing upstream to consider the dynamic
relationships of current, rocks, and holes ahead, much thought is given to
entry: precisely where and at what angle the raft should enter the lead edge
of churning water. The experienced rafter eyes the course ahead, combining

what she sees with what she knows: that Horn Creek Rapid is treacherous at low flow, that Lava Falls is nasty, brutish, and short. There's much to consider before proceeding, but where the current pushes you next and how hard one must pull to avoid capsizing depend a lot on your starting place.

The raft of my education spun wildly into the practice of medicine, a clumsy entry followed by evasive maneuvers. I came from a place of privilege—white suburbia, solid family, excellent schools—but had no idea what I was doing. I wanted to be a doctor but hungered to know much more. As an undergraduate at Washington University in St. Louis, I completed my pre-medical requirements—physics, organic chemistry, and biology—but did lab work in botany and majored in English literature. I grew intoxicated with active knowing—"keying out" the family of a plant from the structure of its flower, tracking an ionic current down the axon of a nerve cell, tracing the complex interactions between intellectual history and literature. The most formative influences, however, weren't ideas but persons: classroom mentors who showed me the "how" of their professions.

Howard Nemerov, the celebrated poet, loved how words play together on the page, how stories unfold, reveal, and puzzle. He once told our class about a graduate student tutorial in which the he and his pupil spent afternoons in his office closely reading and discussing texts. Several weeks into the semester, the student looked up from the page and said, "I see what reading is. It's putting together what you've got with what it says." It was a cry of wonder and recognition, like a scientist discovering where seemingly unrelated facts arrange—aided by theory—into a coherent, beautiful whole.

Ursula Goodenough, a biologist who was memorable for more than her surname, displayed a combination of sensitivity, curiosity, and humility for which I have no other word than "soul." A rigorous scientist and teacher, she initiated undergraduates into the mysteries of molecular biology, each word and gesture testifying that the proper end of science was wonder. She had readily apparent affection, not only for the complexity of organisms, but the fact that they—or anything—existed at all.

Bill Karaikolas, an English professor who loved classroom teaching and barely tolerated academic politics, showed me how to build words into sentences, paragraphs, and essays. I entered his class imagining I already knew how to write. Karanikolas proved me wrong. Being a true teacher, he wasn't satisfied with that. Over the course of a semester, he worked on me like a car mechanic, ripping out a misfiring engine and rebuilding it part by part. By semester's end, his marginal comments on my essays had changed from "Oh my God, no!" to "You've made the best of a bad business," and finally to "This may be finest of the bunch." It was hard-earned praise.

As graduation approached, I applied to medical school *and* graduate programs in English literature. I resembled an indecisive rafter driven by the current towards a huge rock: I could choose my route—rowing hard toward the rocky alley to the right or the standing wave to the left—or let the river choose for me. My middle class parents, who had by then graduated four children from college with one more trailing me, were in no position to fund graduate school in literature, so I applied for scholarships. Not just any scholarships, but big ones like the Rhodes and Marshall, as if I belonged in such heady company. I made a respectable distance through the various selection processes, but none came through. The river chose: I went with Plan B and entered medical school, not even bothering to leave St. Louis.

Washington University presented new students with a first patient beyond our ability to harm: a cadaver of whom we knew neither name nor history. Throughout gross anatomy lab, fellow students gathered at metal tables and confronted the common starting place of modern medical education: a human body, dead. My lab partners, Josh and Elizabeth—who would soon be dead herself, killed in a car accident two months before medical school graduation—pulled back the plastic sheet that covered our cadaver between lab sessions. We carefully inspected the body before starting our dissection—to reach your destination you must know where you're starting from—and made our first cuts with the scalpel in short, ineffectual strokes, less out of squeamishness than legitimate awe and misplaced caution. By semester's end, we'd grown assertive, slicing ligaments with one pass of the scalpel, bluntly separating tissues along fascial planes, tossing scraps in disposal bags like a butcher saving gristle for the family dog. We learned early the principle of medical detachment, coming to see the body before us as material to be mastered, not the physical reality of what once was, like us, a living person.

The materiality of death occupied our attention in gross anatomy lab. It commanded mine so fully I barely noticed Jill, the woman in bright clothes and big earrings stooping over the cadaver at the next table. Had someone prophesied she would be my wife in four years, I wouldn't have believed them. Anatomy lab is no place for romance. Not until second year did we notice one another, become close friends, and fall in love. Then, when lectures grew tedious and hormones untamable, Jill and I would discreetly leave the hall—carefully timing our exits a few minutes apart—and head for the elevator. In a dim basement hallway just outside the animal laboratories, we fell into one another's arms, hungrily kissing, the air ripe with the smell of rodent musk and Purina Rat Chow. For a couple that first met over adjacent cadavers, we shared a nose for romantic settings.

Our class learned the necessity of relying on one another as co-learners, occasional tutors, and consolers. The sheer volume of material, none of it yet involving living bodies, was head-spinning. "Like drinking from a fire hydrant," the Assistant Dean said, promising us that, for those who stayed the course and became doctors, "It doesn't get better; it just gets different." I made plans to temporarily leave medical school for something—anything—less consuming, but didn't follow through. Staying seemed safer than bailing out. The world beyond medicine flickered out the way the countryside below disappears as a plane enters a cloud. I felt my body go soft as my head filled with facts, theories, and disembodied abstractions.

Live patients arrived in third year, the physicality of living bodies providing much-needed context for countless lists memorized and lectures endured. I cycled through the various specialties, trying on each one in turn, sizing them up as possible careers. Self doubt and clumsy hands confirmed that surgery was not for me. I cared for women in childbirth, homeless men in the jaws of psychosis, and frail bodies near life's end. In pediatrics, I found natural comrades in the doctors I worked with and the children we cared for.

Unlike the silent cadavers in gross anatomy lab, patients come with stories. Often, they arrive in existential crisis, when death has ceased to be an abstraction. How should I respond to fellow humans in mortal distress? How much could I care before my emotions limit my capacity to heal? The standard advice is to avoid becoming overly involved with one's patients. There's truth and wisdom in that. A little detachment goes far in difficult terrain. Compassion should serve, not overwhelm, clear-headed decision making.

The most influential defense of physician detachment comes from Dr. William Osler, a nineteenth-century physician widely celebrated as the "Father of Modern Medicine." Osler revolutionized medical education by insisting that students learn at the patient's bedside at least as much as in the lecture hall. Osler helped create the modern system of residency, the hands-on apprenticeship that follows medical school graduation. Regarding detachment, he wrote that the effective physician cultivates two virtues, one bodily and one mental.[1] The bodily virtue is imperturbability, a "judicious measure of obtuseness," a consistently visible distance from patients. The corresponding mental virtue is equanimity, a stoic calm even in the most trying circumstances. Osler never wanted his students to be callous to suffering. He wanted them sufficiently insensible to a patient's pain to deliver appropriate care. Intense feeling clouds the intellect, or so the thought goes.

1. See Osler, "Aequanimitas," in *Aequanimitas*.

While he considered further gentlemanly virtues necessary for the ideal physician, these two stood at the profession's core.

The theory sounded simple, like telling a rafter the safest way to run a river lies in avoiding the holes, but putting simple wisdom into practice is never simple. Only by trial and error over the course of a career does a physician approach Osler's golden ratio of compassion to detachment. In the beginning, one learns by example. The most senior doctor on a medical team—one who has finished his or her education (medical school, residency, and perhaps a fellowship) and supervises trainees—is called an attending physician. An "attending" is the patient's physician of record, the doctor with the final word on team decisions. When the patient wants the straight story, she talks directly to the attending. The attending shows the rest of the team how it's done. At least that's the theory. My attendings offered examples of bedside manner ranging from convivial to wooden. I remember the best by name.

Dr. James Keating, a burly pediatric attending at St. Louis Children's Hospital, had a quick wit and short temper. He cared ferociously for his patients and just as strongly about words. He had little patience for those who proved careless about either. In his own way, he was compassionate, offering counsel and instruction to anyone who shared his unshakeable concern for the patient's welfare. He reserved his wrath for those who took careless short cuts or bent the truth.

When Jill and I left St. Louis for Cleveland, where I did my residency in pediatrics and Jill in obstetrics and gynecology, I met Dr. John Kennell, who studied how to emotionally support mothers and their babies during and after delivery. Tall and thin, Dr. Kennell moved with the lanky ease of Jimmy Stewart. His soft-spoken manner gave patients and students a sense that they were, for the moment, the most important persons on the planet. He often reminded us how different our residency experience was from his. We had complex arsenals of tests and treatments at our disposal, and used them day and night to probe and—we hoped—heal our patients. In his training, residents had much less they could actually do, affording more time to spend in careful physical diagnosis and—wonder of wonders—talking to patients and families. What we had gained through improved means of diagnosis, therapy, and control often displaced, in time and importance, the practice of listening presence.

And there was Dr. Karen Olness, a pioneer in global child health, who taught with economy of words the importance of quiet, attention, and the hard work of listening to what the patient is really saying. Her interests were diverse, ranging from organizing international disaster relief teams to pediatric hypnotherapy, and she threw herself wholeheartedly into each endeavor as if it were her last chance to make a difference. She cared about children, especially those most likely to be overlooked by health care systems already in place, whether in Cleveland or Laos.

The English verb "to attend" can mean to pay attention, to be present to, or to serve, escort, or accompany. The role of attending physician requires considerable knowledge and experience as well as the complex talents necessary to lead and teach by example. What mentors like Keating, Kennell, and Olness taught me is summed up simply enough: they listened, they spoke with care, and they never stopped learning. Under their tutelage, and after years of formal education, I earned the titles "doctor" and "pediatrician." I steered my raft through the early whitewater with mentors to guide me. My credentials said I was ready to be an attending. I didn't feel ready.

* * * *

If my being an attending was all that persuaded Kalene to invite me to a family wedding, there should be many more doctors in this hogan. Far better professionals than I work in the Indian Health Service, men and women who humble me with intelligence, devotion, and tenacity, who patiently turn the dross of inadequate resources into the gold of healthy communities. The trajectory of what I call my career can't compete with theirs. I've been led elsewhere to practices that complement rather than supplant medicine. I became a better doctor on the Navajo reservation. The same goes for my work in Central America and inner city clinics. That part of my education—that "leading out"—came through complex interactions of circumstance, particular people, and grace. I'm a better pediatrician for having been a husband and father, roles at least as challenging as medicine. Marriage (the word for it in Navajo can be translated as "getting used to one another") is, among other things, a shared lesson in patiently attending—and responding—to an always mysterious Other, discovering what's important and letting go of what's not. Parenthood, too. I too long valued thinking and knowing over feeling. I like to imagine I've grown more balanced. I often fail. Like medicine, marriage and fatherhood lead me out of the safety of comforting abstractions into messy ambiguities of human bodies and persons.

I also write things down, capturing that messiness on the page. Writing is a practice of focused attention and response using the available tools, which happen to be words. Words are as lovely and ambiguous as bodies, refusing to bend to the author's will, forever straying from their assigned posts. With words, there's no such thing as triumph, only close encounters with what we meant to say. We try. We fail. We try again.

Words fail to capture the fullness of my wandering journey here, though I recount way stations on the pilgrimage: a Navajo girl dying in an Indian Health Service hospital, the specter of a boy in rural Honduras, the knowing smile of a mother in luminous Guinea brocade, medical cases without remedy. I return to them in memory, less from obsession than desire, as a Talmudic scholar revisits vexing passages in Torah, wrestling with the text in hope of a blessing. They're crucial episodes in a long story, informing and illuminating my life's furthest corners. Like refugees in diaspora, they find surprising ways to communicate in the absence of a common language. They gesture toward something like unity, if never uniformity. My non-medical life and my medical practice inform one another, partners in an ongoing conversation. That conversation somehow led me to the Navajo nation, then away for awhile, and back again, like a probe launched into space to investigate other worlds before returning, however improbably, to earth.

Sitting on the dirt floor of the hogan, I glimpse, however dimly, why my medical lectures, textbooks, and journal articles were necessary but insufficient. I know just enough about Navajo weddings to be sure that, when the bride arrives, the *hatal łii* will sing and tell stories, perhaps remembering with the new couple what First Man and First Woman saw and did as they emerged in this, the glittering world, or how Changing Woman wedded the Sun and gave birth to the Hero Twins. Stories—and the practices that accompany them—are the living heart of tradition. The rabbi and priest, folksinger and novelist, griot and historian all know and inhabit this truth: some things—often the most important—can't be transmitted directly, in so many words. They're best received "slant," to use a word favored by Emily Dickinson.

There is much that medicine must tell directly, unslanted, and unstoried. For some matters, there is no other way. To not know these lessons makes a bad, even deadly, physician. When a diabetic child on an Emergency Room gurney draws deep and labored breaths, it's essential that I recognize the pattern of Kussmaul respirations, a sign of severe acid-base imbalance, part of this girl's critical condition called diabetic ketoacidosis. And when I draw a blood gas to determine how unbalanced the acids and bases in her system have become, it helps to recall the Henderson-Hasselbalch equation—a mathematical description of the acid imbalance I'm witnessing—to respond appropriately. But what I'll also want to know, in order to best help this child, is her story: how long she's had diabetes, how well she controls her sugars, how she became ill this time, what her parents have done to help, and what they're doing, thinking, and feeling right now.

Even more tellingly, when a mother, whose son I've just met, tell me that he's recently lost weight despite a hearty appetite and urinates far more often the usual, I take time, while dipping the boy's urine for glucose to confirm what I already know, to consider what I'll say to his mother. Names are a good starting place for a story. The boy's name is Paul; his mother's is Joy. I could simply give them information: that essential parts of Paul's pancreas are dying, that he'll likely spend the rest of his life taking insulin by one means or another, and that I and my colleagues are about to teach Joy a great deal about diabetes she needs to (but doesn't yet) know in order to care for her son. But to do only that ignores how the three of us—Joy, Paul, and I—are already in a story not of our own making. To offer her no more than information renders me a passionless, if heroic, protagonist, saving her son with my practical knowledge. That's a story, too. Just not a true one.

When I met Joy and Paul in real life one day in my office, I'd already lived through enough stories to do things differently. Yes, I told the Joy I thought her son had new onset diabetes, and I shared some of what would happen during their stay in the hospital. But I said these and other things while also making clear to her that I knew their lives were, from that moment on, irrevocably changed in ways they'd never desired. Beneath the words of her questions about getting to the hospital, I knew she was asking the most urgent and abiding question of any parent: "Will my child be all right?" I shared a brief story or two before sending them down the street to the hospital. There would come time to tell them other important facts.

Stories weave the fabric of my lessons in doctoring. They mark a path to where I am—not simply how I came to be sitting on the dirt floor of a hogan, waiting for a wedding to start, but how I lived into the practice of medicine: the messy, deeply flawed, and beautiful profession I call mine. They aren't "inspirational" in the conventional sense. I have no tales of plucky individuals overcoming vast odds on the road to success. I am forever privileged as a physician, but never more so than when I share another's suffering, however briefly. The most revealing stories travel to places standard medical procedurals dread: where cure is impossible, though the task of caring remains. It's there, where the technologies of control and the specialized knowledge to make it all come out right in the end fail, that I learned profound lessons. These are stories of how I started on the path toward becoming not just a physician, but—in a small, imperfect way—a healer.

Chapter Two

Brian

Cleveland, Ohio

BRIAN DIED IN CLEVELAND on a late autumn night when the sky turned cloudy and tasted of snow. The evening rush in the Emergency Department had ended, but an incoming ambulance radioed ahead with information on an eight year-old boy coming to us from home. His name caught my attention. Not many children share mine. The boy's mother had called 911 less than an hour before, saying her son was confused and too weak to walk. The Emergency Medical Technicians riding in the ambulance described him as alert and coherent, but tired-looking. Was this a true emergency, or a family's panicked response to a child needing sleep? We'd already had several squad runs that night. All those patients had gone home after minimal treatment. I turned to the resident, two years my junior in the medical training hierarchy, who had been listening to the call with me. She'd been in the program more than a year, and I liked working with her. She was competent, calm, and funny—the trifecta of personality traits in a colleague.

"What should we be thinking about with this kid?' I asked, assuming the role of mentor. I was in my first year of a general academic pediatrics fellowship. Far less grand than it sounded, my fellowship served as an educational halfway house between residency and attending, uncertain as I was about leaving the safety of the academy. The resident and I sifted the radio information and began a quick differential—a list of potential diagnoses that could explain the symptoms. It's an important mental practice, a way of surveying the territory at the beginning of a diagnostic hunt to keep the physician from plunging too far down the wrong trail.

"Toxic ingestion," she volunteered, tugging at the collar of her surgical scrubs. "Sure," I said. The boy could have swallowed someone else's medicine, but I pointed out that this would be more likely in a toddler than an eight-year-old. "How about CNS?" she countered, a shorthand term for "central nervous system." CNS injuries range from common events, such as a seizure or concussion, to the rare, such as a childhood stroke. We agreed that we needed more information. More importantly, we needed a look at our patient before we could pursue that.

We were still making our mental list when Brian arrived on a rolling stretcher pushed by the ambulance crew. His eyes were half closed, his head slightly bent forward from a half-sitting position. A white towel draped over his neck and shoulders hid close-cropped hair on the back of his head. With assistance, he stood up and walked to the triage area. There, a nurse asked questions while checking his pulse, respirations and temperature. We sized him up at a distance: a short, thin boy speaking to the nurse in polite, deferential tones. He looked tired, not critically ill.

The nurse rolled him back to an open examining room in a wheelchair accompanied by his mother. Brian flashed a weary grin. His mother, though, looked grave, her eyes hauntingly searching, looking for . . . what? Reassurance? Confirmation she had brought her son to the right place? I'd never seen a face at once so expressive and opaque.

The resident and I glanced at the vital signs recorded on his triage sheet. His pulse and respirations were a little fast, and he had a low-grade fever. I sent the resident in to assess him while I attended to other business. Minutes later, she emerged to tell what she'd learned. Brian had been feeling "under the weather" for days: a nagging cough, sniffles, no fever. He'd eaten poorly. His mother found him that evening slumped over in the bathroom, confused and weak. He denied taking any medicines, pills, or new foods. No recent head trauma; no seizures. He was usually a healthy kid. He now knew where he was and how he had arrived there. The resident told me most of his examination was normal, but he was mildly dehydrated, judging from his dry lips and history of decreased urine output, although his eyes weren't sunken and his capillary refill—the time needed for a healthy pink color to return to the fingertips after firm pressure—was normal. She suggested we start an IV and check some lab tests, including rapid tests of his oxygen and blood sugar. I agreed and let her get started, while I returned to the other patients in the ED, waiting to be seen. I'd soon be in to examine Brian myself.

A few minutes later, the resident was back, looking apologetic. "I've tried several times," she said, "but I can't get his IV started. His veins are hard to find. He may be sicker than I thought. Can you try?"

I went in immediately. Brian eyes were enormous. He trembled on the exam table, his chocolate brown body covered only by a white cloth examination gown, the bed sheet pushed aside in a heap. There were fresh band-aids on both arms and one on the back of his right hand. The room was lit with long ceiling fluorescents, and a gooseneck lamp shone at bed-side, probably placed there during the search for a likely vein. Brian was alone except for the nurse helping with the IV. His mother had reluctantly stepped out to finish some paperwork at the front desk. He looked like he was concentrating hard on something he wasn't ready to share with me. He'd just been stuck several times with a needle and knew I was there to poke him again. I took his right hand, startled by its coolness.

"Isn't it good to know that you're going to be okay?" I asked, a line a wise doctor once taught me, words I've seen restore confidence in children lost in the alien world of hospitals. He turned his head slightly in my direction and may have smiled. I'm not sure. I was already pressing his fingertips to check his circulation when he vomited. It happened suddenly, with no complaint, no retching to warn us. I reached to lift and turn his head a bit so he could clear his mouth, but he stiffened, arched his back, and made an ugly, choking sound. His pupils disappeared behind his upper eyelids.

"He's having a seizure!" the nurse cried.

Some one called for help. The nurse turned Brian's head to the side and suctioned his mouth to clear his airway. All seizures are unsettling, even to those who've seen hundreds of them, but this was more than just a seizure. A rapid assessment told us he was in full arrest: no heartbeat, no breathing, nothing. Brian was dying. Unless we restarted his heart and breath, he would be soon be dead. This was the real thing for which we drilled. With an inflatable bag and mask device, we pushed oxygen into his lungs. His chest rose in response, reassuring us his airway was clear. The resident began chest compressions. Tubes, needles, and medicines appeared from the crash cart. His veins, difficult to find only minutes before, now completely vanished. More than ever, we needed IV access—and quickly. Some medications can be delivered to a patient in arrest by pouring them down a tube placed in the windpipe, but the large amounts of fluid Brian needed could only be given through an IV. We stopped searching for veins in his arms and legs and moved centrally, securing a line in Brian's femoral vein, near his groin. Fluids and medicines flowed while an intern looked for a second IV site. Another resident prepared to place an endotracheal tube. Help began to arrive from other parts of the hospital. Soon two attending physicians, another fellow, and several more residents were gathered in the tiny room. We had no shortage of experience or skill. The room buzzed with well-rehearsed and purposeful activity, but minutes passed without success. Our voices grew increasingly grim. Our movements felt awkward, glacial.

There comes a moment in an unsuccessful resuscitation when the team knows the opportunity to cheat death has passed, that a life is over. We search one another's faces, glance again at the machinery, check the equipment, reassess the patient one last time. Someone may ask if there are any further ideas, anything else to try. The answer is usually "no." I don't remember who finally told us to stop. It must have been an attending, someone with more experience. I hadn't the stomach for it that night.

I also can't recall who claimed the grim task of telling Brian's mother her son was dead. Here things splinter in my memory, shattered by Brian's death. One of the doctors had stepped out to speak briefly with Brian's mother during the "code," gathering information and telling her what we were doing, how we were trying to save her son. Now, from across the hall, I heard a long, piercing wail.

Though I had seen Brian's mother when she arrived, I hadn't spoken with her, much less introduced myself. I made sure to speak with her later, in a quiet room off the ED's main hallway, sharing what little we knew, all we had done, how sorry we were. There was another woman with her, thin and wearing a smart-looking business suit, who kept asking, "But how could he die? How could he die?" I repeated everything I knew. There were no medical answers to her questions. We gave them time with Brian's body, after removing the tubes and bandaging the IV sites. With the lights dimmed and the body covered with a new sheet, he might have been mistaken—in that funeral home banality—for someone sleeping. But there was no chest rise, no breath in his nostrils. His bloodless lips, slightly parted, were pale and still. Again the mother's wail, slow and painful like a knife blade pressed hard against the belly.

I stood silently outside the door; my head slightly bowed, hands crossed before me. The other rooms were already filled with patients who had arrived during our failed rescue attempt. Most of the physicians who had run from other parts of the hospital returned to pressing duties. One stayed to help with the new arrivals. An attending physician directed traffic, restoring order. More of Brian's family gathered, their grieving strangely disconnected from the bustling all around them. I spoke with a minister and again to Brian's mother about necessary forms and the delicate matter of an autopsy, to which she consented. Then the family walked slowly toward the exit, past a waiting room filled with mothers slumped in plastic chairs, where children milled about with mucousy upper lips and Cheeto crumbs pasted to their chins.

Near midnight, after most of the children had been seen, I met the supervisory attending under the glare of an X-ray view box to talk over what had happened, why things went so badly. We spoke of technical matters, things we could alter and control. The cause of Brian's sudden arrest remained unclear. The attending suggested that, early on, we might have placed an intraosseous line, a stiff needle inserted into the bone below the knee, through which medicines and fluids can be given. We agreed it probably wouldn't have changed the outcome, but it was something to remember next time. We wondered what was missing from the history we'd gathered. Nothing Brian's mother said could have made us anticipate the way he died. Save the part about Brian's brief confusion, there was nothing in the ambulance report to hint he was minutes from death. I remembered the feel of his cold hand in mine just before the arrest. What other signs had there been? The attending asked how the rest of the team was doing, especially the resident who had gone in to see Brian first.

"She's all right," I answered, "just shook up about how quickly it happened." We'd all been through the deaths of children, our patients, before. I made a note to talk to her in the morning, reassure her that we were all surprised by Brian's death. Our meeting ended and I walked alone down the long corridor to the garage, pondering questions I knew would defy answers.

What could I have done differently? What had I missed? I've taught emergency pediatric life support, and know the importance of recognizing shock—when circulation doesn't meet the basic needs of the body—as early as possible. Brian's history of confusion and what sounded like a fainting episode now looked like red flags. Why hadn't I examined Brian immediately? In the minutes between Brian's arrival in the Emergency Room and his unexpected death, why hadn't I seen what was coming in time to save his life? Had Brian's determination to walk and talk for himself blinded us to the seriousness of his condition? Medical tradition has it that hindsight is always 20/20 while vision in the moment is forever clouded, but was that just an excuse for errors in judgment? Would things have ended otherwise had I been the first to examine him? Was I to blame? Was there anyone to blame? When a child dies unexpectedly, physicians comb the record for clues and insights, nuggets to keep in one's pocket for the next time. There's something useful to learn from every failure, but failure is also an inexhaustible source of "what ifs?"

An important passage in pediatric residency lies in shedding the North American assumption that the death of children is unnatural, something our ancestors endured, but most of us, thanks to the power of science, only read about in books. Most children—at least in the rich countries of the world's developed North—do, indeed, get better, sometimes *despite* the efforts of their physicians, but pediatric residency ushers young doctors into the veiled world of childhood death. Most of these deaths fall into one of two categories. One sort comes at the end of an overwhelming illness such as childhood cancer or congenital conditions that wither organs and destroy tissues just when children should be reaching toward adulthood. Death is at least theoretically anticipated in any fight against serious illness, often—but not always—permitting doctors and parents time to steel themselves. The other kind of death arrives suddenly, by means unanticipated and often traumatic: traumatic accidents, acute overwhelming illness, or violence. These children arrive in the emergency room already near death, and much effort is compressed in a very short time, as we struggle to reclaim a life. The outcome of a "code" depends on so much beyond our control that we focus on those few things we can change. For a child in cardiopulmonary arrest, death isn't merely possible. It's likely.

What most disturbed me about Brian's death is that he died as I watched, and nothing I did proved capable of reversing that. Why had we— why had I—not been ready? Some doctors stay in that place of doubt, asking the unanswerable again and again the way some patients obsessively touch a scar. Most, however, find ways to shackle the guilt while moving on to the next patient.

The next patient. There's always a next. Sighing, "I'm a professional," the physician walks down the infinite queue of lives, each one demanding to be acknowledged—and rightly so—as utterly unique, the most important person in our world, if only for fifteen minutes of something rather less than fame. A bad cold sends patients and doctors alike to the drug store or medicine cabinet, but when zinc, Vitamin C, and cough syrups fail, we choose between toughing it out or seeing a healer: allopathic, alternative, or otherwise. No matter how vigorously we partner with healers or how thoroughly we tinker with language, assuming the vulnerable role of "patient" (from the Latin *patiens*, to suffer) confesses our human fragility. Even then, like the prisoner in Camus's *The Fall* who's shocked to find he's been sent to a concentration camp, we want to lodge a complaint with someone in authority, "'But, you see sir . . . my case is exceptional!'"[1]

---

1. Camus, *The Fall*, 81.

When I see my physician, I want her empathy and attention. I want her to feel the unique emotional ground from which my banal complaints arise. I don't want her mooning over yesterday's patient. Not on my fifteen minutes. Professionalism demands the physician compartmentalize her doubt, her guilt. New "scientific" management techniques see bad outcomes as problems to be solved. Medical professionals team up to eliminate "systems errors," generate new "clinical pathways," and add to the growing literature of "evidence-based medicine." Such activity restores a sense of control and, we hope, produces a product—an article, report or protocol—others can use to save lives. What unproductive and impractical social feelings remain after all that busyness are banished to the private realm, something between the individual and her counselor.

Sensitive practitioners of modern psychology offer penetrating insights into the human condition, though they find little practical use for the human realities of mourning, doubt, guilt. Mourning, we are told, is something to "work through" in discrete stages of grief. Black holes of doubt that can't be filled by frenetic activity are abandoned, paved over with medication, or passed off to priests and rabbis. And, while conceding that Nazis and pedophiles should feel guilty for their crimes, we're determined to write off less spectacular species of guilt as repressive, atavistic—something best lost in order to become happy, productive citizens. Yes, guilt has been misused historically as a means of social control, but when someone tells me they're "past guilt" the way one might be past puberty, I wonder what other socially significant emotions they numbed along the way. Most healers feel guilty about preventable deaths, particularly the death of children, and any psychological aid offered the wounded healer takes predictable forms. When a medical colleague has something go terribly wrong, sensitive doctors find ways to express concern and offer encouragement: "In a few days, it will be better. We've all been through it. Take your time." I had no trouble keeping busy after Brian's death. There's always the next patient.

Several weeks later, I telephoned Brian's mother about the autopsy report. We arranged a meeting to review it together. I gave her directions to the clinic and reserved a room, clearing my schedule so I would not be interrupted. When she arrived, she seemed much smaller than I remembered. How much more of my memory of that night was distorted? She looked deliberately composed rather than naturally calm, her face still a puzzle. I wondered how she endured a world that continued so undisturbed by the absence of her son. How does anyone awaken—not once, but forever—to such an absence?

We sat down at a table in the half-lit room. I asked if she needed anything before we looked at the autopsy report. She shook her head. I shot a sidelong glance at the box of tissues on the table. A colleague had reminded me to keep one nearby, as if it were always there. I told her again how sorry I was and asked her what questions she had before we began.

"I just want to know," she said, "to understand a little."

"Why Brian died, you mean?" I asked, unsure whether her main interest lay in pathology or philosophy.

"Yes," she said. She looked down at her open hands.

I read the autopsy report slowly and aloud, making sure she understood what the pathologist had found, what had surprised us. At the time of his death, Brian had pneumonia and a pericardial effusion—a bacterial inflammation around the heart. In this light, the history of Brian's cough, however slight, and complaints of weakness and fatigue took on new significance. He had been incubating a very serious illness, perhaps for several days, and the purulent fluid collecting around his heart finally killed him. Had I been the first to examine him, would I have noted the telltale muffled heart sounds of an effusion? Would it have been in time to make a difference? What if Brian had seen a doctor a day earlier? I chose not to explore that just then. I asked instead if, in his last week, he had shown any clues to the severity of his illness? She remembered him as a boy who never complained. Up until his last day, he only said he wasn't feeling well, that he had a cold. Had stoicism been his undoing?

The lab tests we drew in the Emergency Department revealed a very low blood count. Had Brian ever been diagnosed with anemia, sickle cell disease, or any other blood problem? Another blind alley. Brian had received pediatric care in a number of places, whenever his mother could afford it. There were no relatives with sickle cell.

We read over the rest of autopsy together, finding no other surprises. From time to time I paused to study her face, always finding it unreadable. I felt that I, despite all my science, was failing her again. I asked if she could bring us his old medical records, anything that might help flesh out the story. She said she'd gather things together and mail them to me. Then, as if to spare my feelings, she started to bring our meeting to a close, saying she was grateful I had taken the time to meet her, that she appreciated my—and the hospital's—concern and care. She took a tissue as she rose to leave. I stood, too, opening the door to the hallway. I asked if I could show her the way out of the building. She shook her head, saying, "I can manage." I walked with her part of the way, then said goodbye, watching her step slowly, painfully slowly, toward the door. I never saw her again.

Chapter Three

Alice

Tuba City,
Navajo Nation

I DIDN'T FINISH MY fellowship. Some months before I met Brian, I had worked for a month on the Navajo Reservation in Northern Arizona. I returned to the Midwest to complete my education, but my thoughts and my heart remained in the desert. Fellowship had been an experiment, a way to see how I might fit in the province of academic medicine. What I found was a call elsewhere, to stop this formal training and enter the practice. Jill finished her residency in obstetrics and gynecology at the end of the academic year, and we left Ohio in July to work with the Indian Health Service. Our last months in Cleveland were tumultuous, particularly when Jill's pregnancy—our first—was threatened by premature labor. She wanted to prove pregnancy wouldn't interrupt her duties as executive chief resident, and surrendered only when her own obstetrician ordered her on bed rest. Though disappointed, she obeyed, keeping busy with research and administrative work to meet graduation requirements. Then, in the space of a month, we finished training, moved across the country, began new jobs, and added a son.

Will, our blonde-haired Reservation-born Anglo boy, changed everything, including the way I do pediatrics. I'd already learned medicine had to be more than applied book knowledge. Residencies are, after all, apprenticeships, a time to learn from masters of the profession. Parenthood proved strangely similar, though my master was thirty years my junior. Raising

44

ALICE21

a child undermines illusions of control. Many learn how little they truly control long before the arrival of children, but parenthood tutors even the slowest of pupils.

Will did things I hadn't read about in textbooks. He demanded wisdom not found in parenting manuals or advice columns. I carried his lessons with me to clinic, where I grew less dogmatic, less certain that scientific theory neatly corresponded to reality. I disappoint families who want an authoritative—if not authoritarian—doctor, but I've never found it easy to play dictator. Armed with the latest randomized, double-blinded, placebo-controlled trials and sheaves of continuing medical education credits, I step in to the exam room to find a family, messy and uncertain as life itself. Wendell Berry, whose embrace of writing and farming teaches him much about living with uncertainty, says, "medicine is an exact science until applied; application involves intuition, a sense of probability, 'gut feeling,' guesswork, and error."[1]

That last word catches in my throat. Physicians work with bodies, with lives. Until both are perfectly understood—let me know when you've got it—there will be error. But medical errors are of a different order than other mistakes. Most medical errors are, thankfully, small and not life-threatening, but some are fatal. Competence and clinical experience don't preclude error. In leaving my fellowship, I moved into the role of attending, the person of ultimate responsibility in a patient's care. No one supervised my orders now. No one critiqued my decisions unless I asked. I knew my mentors had trained me well, had schooled me in habits that minimize—if never truly eliminate—error, but the powerful tools physicians use to heal just as easily harm, even when used properly. Anyone who's read through a surgical consent form knows the simplest procedure comes with risks. When things go bad, when a patient dies, there may be no end to the self-examination and guilt, even in the absence of identifiable error. I am trained to alleviate suffering and save lives. When a child dies, I feel I've failed.

I don't think about Brian as much as I once did. There are months now when I think I've forgotten him, but he's never really gone. I carry his death like a pocket charm, laying it on the dresser at night with my wallet and keys. And if I ever do forget Brian, I remember Alice.

Alice's father brought her to the Emergency Department on a Saturday night in October, during the Navajo Nation Western Agency Fair. No one volunteers to work the ED on Fair Weekend. Though the Reservation is officially "dry," the Fair brings with it an explosion of alcohol, public drunkenness, hypothermia, car accidents, fights, and sexually transmitted diseases.

1. Berry, "Health is Membership," in *Another Turn of the Crank*, 106.

My first autumn on the Reservation, I was "officer of the day" on fair week-end, the doctor in the ED caring for patients of all ages and infirmities: stab wounds to the chest, truck crashes, and intoxication as well as the usual cuts, colds, and seasonal illnesses. The following year, I made travel plans for Canada to ensure I was unavailable on fair weekend. Things improved when the hospital recruited full time emergency physicians, making officer of the day duty unnecessary. The ED docs saw all patients as they arrived, and the pediatrician on call would come from home to see sick children when needed.

When the call came late that night, it was cloudless and cold. I shiv-ered as I walked through the ED doors. I'd had a busy twenty-four hours, with little time away from the hospital. I hoped this would be quick. The ED doctor had gathered a brief history of Alice's illness, taken a chest X-ray, and ordered some tests. The facts were these: two-year-old Alice had traveled with her family from New Mexico to attend the fair. They'd stayed with relatives in town but planned to head back east that night. She'd had a cold for several days that worsened over the past twenty-four hours. She now had an increasing cough with decreased appetite and activity. Her par-ents said she had felt hot to touch, but hadn't brought a thermometer on the trip. In the ED, her temperature was 100.9 and her breathing was slightly fast, though unlabored.

Most Navajo kids withdraw when examined rather than fight the doc-tor. Alice buried her face in her mother's blouse as I approached, shrugging her shoulders to partially cover her ears. So began the familiar struggle to examine a resistant child. With much help from her mother, I proceeded.

Precisely here in my memories of that night, I run up against some-thing perhaps only doctors can understand. What I see in my mind as I think back on Alice is less how she appeared as a child than the physical findings I noted as her physician. Alice was sick. I was her doctor. I was not after the writer's telling detail, but clues betraying the diagnosis. Surely her face was like so many of the children I'd come to know: reddish-brown with dark, searching eyes. I remember her hair was lighter in color than that of many Navajo children. She didn't look fearful. She likely just wanted me to go away. What I clearly remember, though, is that Alice's mouth was moist, even if she hadn't been drinking fluids well. I lifted her white T-shirt and pressed my stethoscope to her back. Soft crackles and wheezes scat-tered throughout most of her chest, but faded to silence at the upper right. I noted a subtle indentation between and below her ribs with each inspira-tion. She was working harder to breathe than normal. An X-ray removed all doubt: dense whiteness below the shadow of her collarbone, consistent with right upper lobe pneumonia. Pulse oximetry—a sensor attached to her finger—showed a low blood oxygen level: not immediately life-threatening, but too low to send her home.

Her father, however, was adamant about driving the six hours back to New Mexico that night. He'd had a bad experience at our hospital before—something he didn't care to discuss—and wanted his daughter elsewhere. I thought his plan unwise and told him so. He studied me intensely, his right hand drifting up to the rim of his cowboy hat, while I described his daughter's disease, how she needed antibiotics, fluid, and oxygen to help her body get better. Careful to avoid warnings about "what could happen if you don't do as I say," which to traditional Navajo can sound as though the doctor wishes them harm, I described how some children with pneumonia get sicker before our medicines have a chance to work. Children with her condition might take a sudden turn for the worse on a long car ride, far from medical care.

Navajo families sometimes negotiate with the doctor to coordinate treatment with traditional healers, but Alice's father never mentioned it. It was her mother who finally decided, "We will keep her here tonight. When she's better, we take her back home." Grateful for Navajo matriarchy, I busied myself with arranging the admission.

Once on the pediatric ward, I reviewed more fully the story of Alice's illness with her parents, asking many questions. Many of them must have sounded irrelevant to her case. Her father looked incompletely resigned to this annoyance, rarely answering my questions, turning from time to time to his wife as if to ask, "Is this really what you wanted for our daughter?" I believed we were doing the right thing. Even so, I'm a habitual second guesser, forever wondering if I've chosen poorly or missed the obvious.

Doctors are trained to be systematic, asking questions in received patterns so clues aren't missed or diagnoses prematurely discounted. Or so we say. With experience, physicians streamline history taking, screening for pertinent facts, following likely scents. Much of the time we're right, but efficiency has its price. When reviewing a chart at a teaching hospital, the most thorough note may be written by a compulsive medical student who hasn't yet learned what questions are "unimportant." Her note might even yield the ore from which a missed diagnosis is refined.

As it happened, nothing in that night's historical review that night altered my diagnosis. I examined Alice again as her family settled into the hospital room. Little had changed. A clear plastic nasal cannula was taped in place at her nose, supplying oxygen. She was breathing more easily than in the ED, but she looked scared. The admitting nurse that night was Linda, an Anglo with experience in pediatric care and a reputation for speaking her mind. When tensions ran high, she turned blunt, even tactless, but she knew her job and was good with kids. Still, nothing she said or did during her assessment comforted our patient, and the two of us only made matters worse by taking Alice to the procedure room and starting an IV in her arm. She cried in great, breathless sobs, as much, perhaps, from the terror and indignity of being held as from pain. Her father waited in her room, and she quieted only when returned to his arms.

Afterwards, I sat at the nurse's desk to review her admitting orders, which were standard, formulaic. Several other children on the floor that night were being treated for pneumonia. Hogans—traditional eight-sided Navajo homes—are usually heated with smoky wood stoves. Many government-built houses of the four-sided variety also burn wood for heat. In October, desert nights turn cold, and kids were back in school, so respiratory illnesses were common. Asthma and pneumonia often brought children into the hospital. Alice seemed much like the others, and I looked forward to her going home in a day or two.

"Brian." Linda called from Alice's room.

"What?" I answered dully, not ready to leave my chair.

"This IV's not working."

I was up in a moment, intent on proving Linda wrong. It had been a difficult IV to start. I didn't want to stick Alice again so soon. IVs are tricky and delicate: a thin teflon cathether thrust into a superficial vein, held in place with adhesive tape and hope. In young children, we secure these contraptions with soft armboards, padding, gauze and plastic cups, but the complex geometries of tube and vein can go awry even as we tape and reinforce, destroying in seconds a quarter hour of work.

While Linda steadied Alice's forearm, I gently removed the tape and played with the catheter, watching carefully for the IV fluid to start flowing again. It never did. There was nothing to do but pull it out, stanch the bleeding, and start over on another vein. Linda left to ready the procedure room while I explained the situation to Alice's father. He looked unhappy but resigned. Once again, he remained at Alice's bedside while we took her, wailing pitifully, to the procedure room. We recruited the medical assistant to help us and I tried to start her IV again.

And again.

And again.

I'd started IVs for years—there was no one awake and in the hospital that night better at it—but Alice's body rejected my every assault. I could feel the slight give as needle and catheter pierced the venous wall, followed by a bluish swelling signaling a ruptured vein. She gained three new bruises, but no IV access. Three times in one sitting is all I'll attempt unless access is critical. I pressed again on her fingertips, counting the time it took for color to return as I released: less than two seconds. Alice wasn't in shock. She didn't need an intraosseous line. IV antibiotics were ideal in her case, but I could prescribe a workable alternative: antibiotics injected into her thigh. Each shot would hurt and the medicine would be absorbed slowly, but this seemed a better choice than torturing a two-year-old at one a.m. At sunrise, I or someone else might have better luck.

I explained our change of plans to Alice's father, who sat silently in his chair, his hat now resting in his lap. He stared at me as I spoke, his eyes filled with skepticism. I had hoped to relieve his doubts about the hospital. There was little chance of that now. Embarrassed and angry at myself, I returned to the nurses' station and rewrote the antibiotic order. I hoped it would be the last task of the night. I had been through far worse in residency, but I'd been a younger man then and more tolerant of long hours.

On my way out, I stopped at Alice's room. She was drowsy but awake, her hair swept to one side. Her father had settled in a chair, the hat back on his head and tilted forward, almost covering his eyes. Except for the steady bubbling of oxygen, all was quiet. I walked down the darkened hallway past the mural of Tu-tu-vi-neh, the Hopi boy who became an eagle; past the painting of the Navajo grandfather in his hogan; past the empty, unmarked morgue. At last out the door, I stepped into darkness full of stars and pinyon smoke. The fairgrounds glowed in the distance. I would be off duty in the morning, when Steve, my colleague, would take over the ward. By the time I walked home and crawled in bed, Alice should have received her first an-tibiotic dose. We would both feel much better by dawn.

Two hours later, the pager squawked on my bedside table. I groped for the phone. It was Linda. "Alice's breathing harder," she said.

"Does she look like she's in distress?" I asked.

"No. She's sleeping right now. She was taking clear liquids by mouth with no trouble. No fever, no other changes. She just seems to be working harder."

Not fully awake yet, I asked for clarification: "You mean her breathing?"

"Yes."

"Do you think I need to come in?"

A brief pause. "No. Respiratory therapy's been busy on the adult side, but he's here now and thinks he can make her more comfortable."

We agreed Linda would call again if Alice did not improve. I hung up the phone, stared at the ceiling and, as with most nighttime calls, commenced second-guessing. The telephone and thermometer are two-edged swords in clinical medicine, providing tantalizing—if incomplete—information, simultaneously reassuring and disturbing. A pediatrician often relies on a third person for the patient's story: a parent, a grandparent, a baby sitter. Someone other than the patient describes the symptoms, says what they want done. I had a good team on tonight, though, and I had no doubt they would call me in if things worsened.

Linda paged again forty-five minutes later. "She's definitely tugging now."

I said I'd be right in. Jill, pregnant with our second child, stirred in bed but didn't awaken. I threw on some clothes and tiptoed past Will's room, grabbing a denim jacket on my way downstairs. Our house was five minutes on foot from the hospital. The brisk walk guaranteed I'd be alert by the time I reached the pediatric unit. The night was icy black without hint of sunrise. The fairground had lost its nimbus of light.

I entered the hospital through the ED. A man snored on a gurney in the darkened examination room, fluid slowly dripping through an IV into a vein in his right arm. The waiting area was vacant. Through dim hallways, I walked past labor and delivery, past silent operating rooms, and onto the pediatric unit, where only Alice's room and the respiratory therapy office spilled light onto the hallway floor.

I could see from her doorway how much Alice had worsened. She was breathing faster and with prominent retractions—using the muscles above her collarbone to help move air in and out of her lungs. Somewhere during the past two hours, her parents had traded places. Alice's mother reached across the bed to console her daughter, who rolled back and forth on her haunches as if refusing to awaken. Round the mother's neck hung a simple handmade necklace, a turquoise stone swaying with every move. Her burning gaze turned on me in silent interrogation. I told her what little I knew: Alice was sicker, and we would do our best to find out what was going on while our medicines did their work.

I reached for my stethoscope, rubbing the diaphragm against my shirt to brush away the night chill. With her mother to support her, I examined Alice's chest, watching the girl's increased work of breathing, percussing her lung fields with a brisk snap of the wrist, listening carefully front and back. Except for her right upper lobe, she had good breath sounds and no more wheezing. Her pulse and respirations were fast, even for a young child. I pressed her fingertips and counted the seconds until the color returned: capillary refill was normal.

Often during night visits to the hospital, I grow conscious of how slowly I think. Perhaps no one else notices. Maybe it's only subjective time distortion. I tremble in fits of mental sluggishness, as if waiting for the magic eight ball's advice to float into view. It's not so much fatigue but the loneliness of these fugue states that disturbs me. With no one there to bounce ideas off of, I have to figure things out for myself, beginning with the most basic questions: What's going on with my patient? What's the story I've stumbled into, and where am I in it? It's then I rummage silos of memory for anything similar in my medical experience. If the long, beastly hours of residency training have any payoff, it's when I must cut through the mental fog with systematic thought: What's the problem? What must I know in order to respond effectively? How can I best obtain that information?

I pondered the situation, spoke briefly with Linda and the respiratory therapist, and set to work. I remember the struggle to get an arterial blood gas, or ABG, from her wrist. This would tell me how effectively she was getting oxygen to her tissues and how well she was ridding her body of carbon dioxide. Arteries are more protected and more pain-sensitive than veins. I've performed countless arterial punctures in my career, but I've never liked doing them. Alice sobbed while her mother watched me attempt—and fail—to get the proper sample. Eventually, I settled for second best: a simpler but less useful venous blood gas coupled with a finger probe to monitor blood oxygen saturation.

Was I doing Alice any good? Not only was her body acting in unexpected ways, but I now seemed unable to make my own body do as I wished. I was failing at simple procedures I had done countless times before. Self-doubt was rising in floodwaters, and I had to stay on task or be washed away. My patient was ill. There was too much to do.

There was the usual grumbling unpleasantness with Kee, the nighttime X-ray tech who was never happy to be called in from home. There was more second guessing as I reviewed my admitting orders, puzzling over what I might have missed, rethinking antibiotic choices. Alice's parents constantly hovered at the edge of my awareness and I returned to her mother frequently to report progress, however small. Despite my difficulties, I was increasingly thankful Alice hadn't left town with her family. I pictured her in the family pickup, worsening with each mile on the darkest, loneliest roads in the lower forty-eight states. Yet how much better was she doing here? The lab tests gave me confusing results. Only one thing was clear: I hadn't made her better. Feeling ever more a failure, I walked to the nurses' station and called Steve, the pediatrician who would soon relieve me.

Unflappable and clear-headed, Steve is a physician I don't mind asking for advice and a friend I hated to disturb. I began to explain the case over the phone but Steve stopped me and, without being asked, volunteered to come in. He had worked on the Reservation longer than I, and knew how valuable an extra pair of eyes and hands could be when things aren't going well.

I was in Alice's room when I heard the familiar rhythm of Steve's limping gait, the result of childhood hip disease. He's spent much of his

life proving the insignificance of his injury, and the concentration and per-
sistence he brings to downhill skiing and rugged backcountry treks carry
over to his work as a doctor. He was already warming his stethoscope in
his cupped hands as he entered the room, but we quickly stepped into the
hallway where I could tell him the story. In truncated form, I recited the
essentials of a standard medical presentation: history, physical exam, laboratory data, and medical course since arrival in the hospital. We squinted at
her X-rays in the hallway light. Steve then examined Alice while I waited at
the doorway like a medical student watching the professor. Despite Alice's
worsening illness and the indignities of the night, she was still alert and
reasonably cooperative, sitting by her mother, eyes trained on Steve, wary
of this latest threat.

When Steve finished his exam, we excused ourselves and once again
stepped into the hallway to talk. Steve said he couldn't find anything I
had missed. Simply having someone I respect tell me, "You're doing what
I would do," is valuable reassurance, confirmation that I'm not harming
someone through sheer boneheadedness. She would need an IV, though,
not only for antibiotics, but for fluids too, since her increased heart rate
could be a response to dehydration. We agreed to try another blood gas,
the results of which could be decisive. Her labored breathing could not be
sustained for long, and if, despite her efforts, she did not effectively rid her
body of carbon dioxide, we would need to place her on a ventilator. That,
in turn, would force further action. Our hospital had a small intensive care
unit with room for three or four adults, but Alice would need specialized
pediatric care in Phoenix, five hours south by ambulance. A medical air
transport team, including a flight nurse and respiratory therapist, was the
only reasonable way for her to get there: an involved, time-consuming process. I silently considered what Alice's father might say about a proposed
transfer to Phoenix, noting that I hadn't seen him since my return to the
hospital. Alice's mother was still on the pediatric unit, and if we came to the
point where Alice had to travel, we would not only need parental consent,
but a family member to go with her.

IV, fluids, blood gas, possible intubation and transfer. I mentally tallied
the tasks before us.

"How do you want to divide the work?" I asked Steve. He responded
with characteristic generosity, pointing out that he was due to begin duty in
less than an hour, that he was already awake, dressed, and in the hospital,
and that he could take over for me now. I felt torn: determined to see Alice
through her illness, yet exhausted by a long and frustrating night. Linda,
at the end of her twelve-hour shift, was already turning over her patient
to the new nursing crew. They were hard-working and used to long hours,

but few things make me feel more fatigued than a team of fresh faces at the start of their day, ready for patients who have kept me up all night. Leaving now seemed, in the body-denying machismo of medicine, weak, as if I were placing my body's need for sleep ahead of my patient's recovery.

"What if you need to intubate her?" I asked, anticipating the delicate process of placing a sick child on a ventilator.

"She's old enough that I'll probably call anesthesia," Steve replied. "You don't need to stick around for that."

"How about I at least start the IV?" I asked. Steve was insistent, though, and at last I surrendered him the floor, "signing out" the patients on the unit with quick summaries of diagnoses and conditions.

Even then, I lingered a bit, reviewing the night to make certain I hadn't forgotten something crucial. Labor and delivery was quiet when I told the nurses there that Steve was taking over. I returned to the pediatric unit and checked on the other patients, all of whom had—thankfully—spent an uneventful night. When I stopped at her room, Alice was still working at each breath, her shoulders gently heaving as she sat in her mother's lap. Strings of dull hair clung to her forehead. Her blanket had fallen to the floor. I told Alice's mother I was leaving for the day and made sure she had met Steve, her daughter's new doctor. She had no questions for me.

Fragile dawn yielded to brilliant morning as I walked home. A lone raven cackled in flight past the cottonwood tree by the abandoned hospital airstrip. Jill was up with our son when I entered the house. Eight months pregnant, she had once again struggled with premature labor, but we were closing in on her due date, and—with her doctor's permission—she was increasingly active. Looking up from the book she was reading to Will, she asked me, "Who's been keeping you up all night?"

I sat down on the couch beside them and told Jill the story while Will crawled over to give me a hug. Steve had been right. As much as I wanted to solve the mystery, it was better for me to be home, leaving Alice's care in his competent hands. So close to the birth of our next child, it was good to be together, just us three.

It's been a blessing these many years, not having to explain to my wife what it's like to be a physician. Jill listened patiently, gave me a hug, and we set about making breakfast: eggs with orange juice and mugs of coffee. We talked while eating; lingering over the crumbs long after Will finished and left his place. Physically drained from a busy call duty, I was content with my good fortune. Jill rose to clear the table, and I was thinking about sitting down with the Sunday paper when my pager crackled: "Come to pediatrics, stat! Come to pediatrics, stat!"

I don't know how other physicians feel about emergency calls, but I've never found them as exciting or glamorous as they appear on television. I usually hope someone's overreacted, that my presence is already unnecessary when I arrive. Will, playing alone on the floor, startled as I grabbed my jacket and headed out at a run. Entering the pediatric unit through the back door, I could hear Steve giving directions in a firm, steady voice. Alice's room was packed, an air transport team—who must have recently arrived by plane from Flagstaff or Phoenix—bunched outside the doorway. The flight-suited crew looked out of place, uncertain what to do, their wheeled stretcher still inside the room, beyond reach. From the door, I saw the head nurse doing chest compressions, while the respiratory therapist was forcing oxygen through a tube in Alice's mouth. Steve was directing another nurse to give a dose of epinephrine by IV. What little I could see of Alice's skin was gray and flaccid, like soft candle wax. I guessed at some of the morning's events: an ominous blood gas result, intubation by the anesthetist, a call to the transport team. But at the crucial moment, when Alice was being readied for her flight, something very bad must have happened.

"I'm here," I called to Steve as I pushed forward to the door. "What do you need me to do?"

Steve half smiled, half grimaced and said, "We were getting her ready to draw a blood gas before she left when she arrested, and I don't know why."

"ET tube's OK?" I asked, wondering if it had moved and was no longer ventilating her lungs.

"Anesthesia placed it and the chest film showed it in good position. It's taped in the same position as then. I just checked her breath sounds and they sound equal."

I borrowed his stethoscope and listened. Air movement was strong and symmetric with each forced breath. During a brief pause in chest compressions, we looked at the heart monitor—no beat, no electrical activity at all.

"Resume compressions," Steve called, and the two of us recited possible cardiovascular catastrophes to explain what we were seeing. Then, as methodically and quickly as possible, we addressed those we could change. We suctioned her endotracheal tube and checked its placement with a laryngoscope: the plastic tube passed, as it should, through glistening white vocal cords. We needled both sides of her chest to rule out life-threatening lung collapse. We used the defibrillator three times to restart her heart, but without success. We carefully advanced a needle from the notch below her breastbone to relieve any fluid or air collection around her heart. With each pause in chest compressions, we checked for a heartbeat, or any electrical activity at all. Again and again, there was none.

"Any other ideas before we stop?"

No one spoke. The nurse doing chest compressions turned her face to Steve, ready for orders.

"Stop compressions."

Alice was dead.

Little more than a century ago, the death of children was commonplace. For the Navajo, for whom the benefits of modern sanitation, electricity, and modern medicine were slow in arriving, appallingly high child mortality outlasted the Second World War. In parts of what we now call "the developing world," as if referring to another planet, early childhood remains a charnel house. Yet, for those fortunate enough to live today in the rich countries of the global north, a child's death comes as a shock, a rupture of what we take to be normal. And so it seems, arriving for most of us more often in news of mass shootings and traffic accidents than in the intimacy of a face-to-face encounter in a single room.

No pediatrician I know, not even those who work in the remotest locations or most dire circumstances, grows accustomed to death, however frequent its appointments. Yet we have all seen children die, reminding even the slowest learner that no one escapes the biology's iron law: all that lives must one day die. In the sudden quiet of a hospital room, we were—all of us—reminded once again.

Steve turned to those who had participated in our unsuccessful attempt to save Alice and softly said, "Thank you, everyone." He stepped out to speak to the flight crew, thanked them for coming, and wished them a safe flight home. The head nurse began to clean up piles of debris left behind: paper, gloves, syringes, soiled towels. Another nurse removed the tubes and wires still connected to Alice's body. Her hair hung in wild clumps, a piece of white tape clinging to several strands falling over her right cheek. Her hands were limp and motionless, like a doll waiting to be picked up. Her chest was finally still. No one could mistake this for sleep. Somewhere in the last few minutes the sensible matter of a person had ceased, by linguistic convention, to be "Alice," and had become "Alice's body." On one side of that divide, we struggled to save her life. Now we readied the body for her parents' grief.

Here again, memories fall apart. Odd, how my vision fails when a patient's death smashes memory's lens. Surely we sat with Alice's mother, told her the whole distressing story. Why can't I remember any of that? I do recall, without images, as if someone had to tell me, that Alice's father could not be found, that he had left the hospital sometime that morning. I remember talking with Steve, the two of us without a specific explanation for Alice's death. I remember feeling drained as the entire team wordlessly returned to work, the day ahead demanding brevity of our sorrow.

The morning had grown warm by the time I left the hospital. The neighborhood was stirring, people on their way to church or out walking the dog. The world would go on without Alice, and I was too exhausted to dwell on unanswerable questions. I walked home in a gray haze of failure. Jill and I silently held each other awhile, as I had done one morning when Jill returned in a similar fog of numbness and fatigue, slump-shouldered and stunned from unexpectedly losing a young mother whose complicated labor went terribly awry. We both knew from experience that, at such times, facts are less important than a knowing touch or a cup of hot tea. She ordered me to bed, and I dozed off and on, awakening in the early afternoon unrefreshed but unable to sleep any longer.

I pulled on my clothes and came downstairs. Jill was sitting at the dining room table watching Will through the window as he played in our tiny backyard. She asked if I was hungry and brought me something to eat as I halfheartedly scanned the Sunday paper. We spoke a little more about Alice, then agreed we should head out to the fair and salvage something of the day. We would all get outside on what was clearly a gorgeous fall afternoon, and I might be able to get my mind off of Alice. Jill wanted to find some presents for Christmas, and any vendors still there would be selling at a discount.

Jill drove to the fairgrounds, and we walked up the dirt road to the sales area, Will riding in a carrier on my back. Many booths were already vacant. The jewelry and crafts still on sale were the sort we could find at the weekly flea market in town. Paper trash and plastic bottles were piled next to overflowing garbage cans sporting the banner: "We protect the earth, our mother." I was about to suggest we head home when we saw Linda walking with her Hopi boyfriend, who also worked at the hospital. They walked over to me and we said quick hellos before she asked, "So how did that girl do?"

I'd forgotten Linda left before I turned things over to Steve. It was clear she hadn't heard the news. When I told her the story, she winced and buried her forehead in her boyfriend's chest. We all stood in silence awhile before she turned back to me and said, "Well, the next time I call you in the middle of the night, I'll be sure to drag your ass out of bed."

Was she making an accusation? Startled, I studied her face, but it had lost none of its apparent sympathy. Her boyfriend looked surprised at her comment, too. I waited to hear if she had more to say, but that was all. I hadn't the energy to pursue it. We said awkward good byes, and I went to find Jill, who had drifted away to look at turquoise jewelry. Linda never talked to me about Alice again, and if she had concerns about my actions that night, I never heard them.

We never learned what Alice died of. There was no autopsy. Navajo custom precludes touching or taking anything from a corpse. Traditional

Navajos bury a body before sunset on the day the person dies. By the time I returned to the hospital Monday morning, there was no evidence Alice had even been there, save X rays, lab data, and a medical record mostly in my handwriting.

On morning rounds, I recounted the story for my pediatric colleagues, with Steve picking up from the time I turned the unit over to him. He told how he had given Alice some intravenous fluid, but without improvement in her breathing or heart rate. Over the next hour, she rapidly worsened, requiring ever-higher amounts of oxygen until it was clear she needed to be intubated. When the anesthetist passed the tube into her trachea, it filled with blood-tinged froth, suggesting a build up of fluid in her lungs, a serious condition called adult respiratory distress syndrome. Steve had been in contact with an excellent pediatric intensive care specialist before and after the transport team's arrival, and did everything he recommended. Alice's arrest began abruptly, when everyone believed her ready for transport. The flight nurse had been gently rolling her to the left when her heart simply stopped.

Another pediatrician shared what he'd heard from a family member before they left on Sunday. Apparently some of Alice's extended family, including her grandfather, gathered at the hospital while her condition was worsening. A Navajo grandfather, or *chei*, is a figure of much respect and affection, with a close bond to his grandchildren. Alice's *chei* had reportedly stood outside her room that night, watching through the large glass window. At some point, he abruptly told the family that he'd seen Alice's *nilchi*—her breath—leave her body, and that she was going to die. That's when he left. Perhaps Alice's father left then, too. I don't know.

Nor do I know whether anyone remembers the story as I do. Steve dictated Alice's hospital summary a few days after her death, in which he describes speaking to "the parents and grandparents" about the benefits of an autopsy. Did the men come back later, or am I confabulating their disappearance at the time of death? When I phoned Steve eight years after the fact, he couldn't answer that question, but it didn't take him long to recall other details. He knew her pneumonia was "right upper lobe," and remembered needling her chest in the final moments. Over the phone, though, I sensed in him none of the emotional confusion still roiling inside me. Steve is a passionate man and compassionate physician, but whatever he was feeling then about Alice's death hid beneath professional detachment, making him a better clinical scientist than I'll ever be. As we talked, he was already comparing Alice's story to other unexpected pediatric deaths on the Reservation. Steve has an eye for statistical trends and clusters, epidemiological hints which, if pursued, may save lives. Even the hospital summary ends by enumerating and carefully considering possible explanations for her cardiac arrest. I, unfortunately, am dogged by less useful, more personal questions.

Should I be? When a case review is complete, shouldn't a physician move on, equipped with lessons learned from the regrettable experience? Wouldn't a colleague tell me to "forgive myself" or "cut some slack"? Physicians rarely tell one another how they feel about a patient's death. Most bring back the dead only in rare, unguarded moments, over a late night beer. So why mull over Brian and Alice? Why write about them?

William Carlos Williams's short story, "Jean Beicke," describes the death of a young girl in the 1930s. Antibiotics, which weren't available for most of Williams' career, might have saved the eleven-month-old in the story, but that's not the point. Williams, who refused to cloak his feelings in psychological pieties, describes the wretched conditions of children abandoned on the pediatric ward and wonders why the hospital staff works so hard to save them. He chides the pediatric nurses for lavishing attention on the least promising cases, suggesting they've saved girls like Jean for life as cheap prostitutes.

I've met doctors who talk that way, caricatures of Williams at his harshest, though only a few—I hope—are as cynical as they sound. Most, like Williams, feign callousness to camouflage affection for patients whose lives are often nasty, brutish and short. Williams's spare storytelling, his careful attention to "the pale sort of blue" of Jean's eyes, and his raw joy in watching the girl devour her meals, reveal his heart. At one point he admits, "we all got to be crazy about Jean,"[2] and when, after Jean's death, he tells the otolarygologist that saving her life would have been pointless, it's clear Williams would give anything to have her back.

In a way, he did bring her back, since we would know nothing of her brief, unhappy life except for Williams's story. He knew where the juice of a story flows, and revealed to his readers his complex feelings about a dying girl. She got under his skin, as Brian and Alice got under mine. Williams—who always maintained that medicine nourished his writing—had to scratch that itch. Now, in a less artful way, I scratch mine. It diminishes Williams's accomplishment to pretend he wrote his story as therapy or catharsis. It doesn't work that way for me. No matter how much I write, Alice remains—dead, but not gone.

She was still with me, months later, when we took a family camping trip to Southern Utah. Jill and I hoped to briefly escape the worries of the hospital, but in the days before we left, the Indian Health Service reported a cluster

2. Williams, "Jean Beicke," in *The Doctor Stories,* 73.

of deaths in young, healthy residents of the eastern half of the Reservation. The victims' initial symptoms resembled influenza—fever, chills, and head-ache—though their condition rapidly worsened, leading to adult respiratory distress syndrome and death. There were as yet no clear risk factors for the disease, and the cause, believed to be infectious, was undetermined. We couldn't know it then, but this was the beginning of the Hantavirus outbreak in the Southwest, an epidemic that would kill several more that summer be-fore the previously unknown virus was identified. The sudden appearance of a new, fatal illness brought with it the usual combination of fear and ugliness: news outlets called it a "Navajo disease," trips and cultural exchanges with off-reservation institutions were suddenly canceled without explanation, and nasty jokes made the circuit. Most of that, I'm sure, arose more out of igno-rance than malice, but it was disturbing to see and hear. By fall, the epidemic was over, the virus identified, and most of the public unpleasantness past. I still wonder, though, if Alice might have been an early case of the epidemic. There's no way to know that now: no postmortem data, no serum saved in which to look for antibodies. Nothing but unanswerables.

As for our camping plans that spring, Jill and I wondered whether we should go. No one could say yet if the apparent cluster of deaths was an epidemic or coincidence. At the time, there had been no case reports from Utah, where we were headed. Jill and I knew too much for our own peace of mind. There was something indefinable to worry about, an amorphous bogey at once as real and theoretical as nuclear annihilation. Finally, given the choice between helplessly worrying at home or in one of our favorite places in the world, we chose to go.

We drove to Cigarette Spring, a favorite campsite perched at the edge of a mesa, where fragrant juniper-pinyon forest gives way to immense vis-tas, deep quiet, and splendid isolation. In all our visits there, I recall meeting only two other humans. We arrived alone, set up camp and began to explore.

The spring weeps from a fractured rock face, collecting in muddy pools and potholes in the rock at the head of a small side canyon of the San Juan River. After a heavy summer rain, water from the spring pools may run all the way to river level before evaporating or heading underground. The previous six months had been unusually wet, and there was more flowing water there than I'd ever seen.

Dozens of black tadpoles swam in nearby shallow potholes, squirming against each other like rush hour commuters at a subway station. After a desert rain, frogs emerge from underground dormancy around lakes, ponds and potholes to engage in shoreline bacchanals full of thrumming male choruses and spirited coupling. Soon enough, they return to the mud and estivate, a hibernation-like state safeguarding them through long droughts.

These tadpole masses before me now, conceived in amphibian orgies, were racing to maturity before the pool evaporated. Their prospects looked grim. In some of the pools, tails and upper bodies were already exposed to the air. Soft mud at the periphery showed how high the water had been only days before. The question was not whether some might die before they could breathe out of water, but whether any would survive at all.

Things could change suddenly, of course. Rain might come any time, replenishing pools and launching another raucous fertility ritual, but the skies were cloudless, and the June drought was fast approaching. I could play savior and add some of our water as token reparation for the relentless human assault on desert wildlife, but to what end? This drama of maturation vs. dehydration was playing out in water pockets throughout the Colorado Plateau. The frogs that laid the eggs from which these tadpoles hatched slept underground, doing what their ancestors did for millennia, what they do to survive as a species.

It's nearly impossible to reflect on such things without drifting into anthropomorphism and exposing the metaphorical scaffolds of human reasoning. We impose human experience onto non-human animals as different from us as tadpoles. It's treacherous territory, and rigorous thinkers dismiss most of it out of hand. If frogs fear death, how would we know? Other mammals exhibit behaviors interpreted as mourning their dead, but humans sustain, through culture, elaborate and varied expressions of grief. Which might explain why stumbling upon a graphic depiction of life's fragility—however foreign that life appears—invites us to pause, reflect on our own fragility and lack of control.

I don't know how long I crouched there, studying the strange black colonies, now motionless in the shadowy rock cleft, my mind reaching back to the short lives and sudden deaths of Brian and Alice, their grieving parents, and my clumsy attempts at professionalism. How absurd for tadpoles to trigger such a reverie. I felt a rising sense of shame, having caught myself wallowing in sentimentality. Or was it a realization that, having died in my presence, these children—and others—follow me like ghosts, trespassing on my awareness at the least provocation? I'm not attracted to the occult. I don't go in for poltergeists and channeling. I know how the brain reifies anxiety, incarnates fear. But at the risk of further compromising my professional status, I confess hoping that whatever spirits—real or imagined—that may shadow me remain benign. In any case, I've learned to live with them. If they shape my practice, it's through the cautionary tales they tell. They remind me of my limits, the things I don't know. When I want to dismiss my failures, they withhold their consent.

I was still in my distracted crouch when Will, not quite four years old, found me. "Daddy," he said, looking down from the rock overhang above the spring, "We were looking for you and I was calling, but you didn't answer. What are you doing?"

I didn't say a word. Instead, I stood, gathered him in my arms, and hugged him tightly. It's a game we both loved to play, seeing how long he could stand my bear hug before telling me to relax my grip. This time, though, he grew alarmed at my ferocity.

"Daddy, you're squeezing me."

But just then, I couldn't hold him tight enough.

Chapter Four

Losing Control

Tuba City, Navajo Nation

THANKSGIVING MORNING SUNLIGHT SLANTED through bare cottonwoods as Peter, our eleven day-old son, wailed from his bedside crib. He'd filled the prior evening with crescendoes of fussiness, periods of fitful sleep, and equally fitful attempts at nursing. I sprawled in bed, unrested, unhappy, and troubled. Jill placed Peter to the breast again, where he squirmed and nibbled, finding no comfort.

"He feels hot," Jill said through tears of frustration. She held our son in her arms, rocking him tightly against her chest, willing him back to sleep.

Frustrated myself, and determined to prove Peter's temperature was normal, I rose to fetch the thermometer from the bathroom. I lubricated the thermometer bulb and took Peter's rectal temperature, prompting new shrieks of distress. Two minutes later, I held the thermometer to the light and squinted through the glass for the tip of the red column.

101.2. Not what I was hoping for. I rubbed my eyes and peered again.

101.2.

I shook the thermometer, rinsed and relubricated the bulb, and took Peter's temperature a second time.

101.3.

All at once, I was fully awake, aware of my consciousness splitting in two, physician's mind and father's heart falling from one another like the lapels of a heavy coat unzipping. My pediatric training turned to data and clinical pathways, telling me precisely what needed to be done and why.

Fevers in babies under two months of age are worrisome because fever is a nonspecific sign of anything from the effects of too many blankets on a hot summer day to a life-threatening bacterial illness. What's more, newborns don't fight certain infections well. When a young infant has a real fever—not one caused by overwrapping, for example—the likely cause is a viral illness, such as a cold, from which the baby suffers no lasting effects. But some viral illnesses and almost all bacterial infections are dangerous in babies, often leading to pneumonia, blood and kidney infections, or meningitis. These life-threating conditions may start while the baby still looks quite good, with little more than fever to suggest something's wrong.

Faced with this uncertainty, pediatricians treat fevers in the very young with great caution. After taking a thorough history and performing a physical exam, the doctor orders a number of tests, including cultures of the blood, urine, and spinal fluid. Then the baby is given intravenous antibiotics until the time—usually thirty-six to forty-eight hours later—negative culture results rule out the presence of serious bacterial illness. If the cultures are negative—far and away the usual outcome—antibiotics are stopped and the baby goes home with mother, exhausted from a hospital stay but otherwise well. If, however, the cultures reveal a bacterial cause, there will be more tests to come and days more of antibiotics until the episode is declared over. With prompt diagnosis and appropriate treatment, many, but not all, infants with serious bacterial illness go on to full recovery.

I knew all this intellectually, the way I know capitals of states, but my heart ran wildly elsewhere, desperate to protect my infant son from needles, X rays, and IV medicines. I'd done enough "sepsis workups" on babies to know how little the patient appreciates the attention. My first, unspoken response to my discovery of Peter's fever was to blame myself for using the thermometer at all. I imagined for a moment that ignorance might have magically insulated him—and us—from harm. Then I remembered babies from my residency whose fevers had been neglected before hospitalization. Some ended up neurologically devastated. Some died. This was no time for magical thinking.

I was learning, from the inside this time, how to ask the parent's universal question: Will my child be OK? That's what a doctor friend of mine asked the day his daughter was diagnosed with new-onset Type 1 diabetes. My friend takes care of many children and adults with the disease, he knows its course and complications, he's up to date on the latest treatments and research, but when his own child fell ill, his first words to the treating physician were, "Is she going to be OK?"

I had entered my own desert of unknowing, the abstractions of professional practice swept aside by the reality of my son's illness. I knew Peter would most likely be fine. For my colleagues at the hospital, he would be another hot baby with a viral infection all but certain to resolve on its own. I also knew it could be otherwise, and I knew what must happen to rule out impending catastrophe. In the country of affections, the power of knowledge threatens to sink of its own weight like a fortress in a bog.

I looked at my son in my wife's arms, his soft black hair tousled, his mouth alternately pouting and grimacing, his arms and legs grappling for comfort. This was intolerable. My head and heart zipped back together, and I said to Jill in my best imitation of calm, "We're taking him to the hospital."

* * * *

When new parents come to me with their firstborn, I congratulate them, take a history, examine the baby, offer anticipatory guidance, and answer as many questions as I can. I understand that they, like me, want to know their child is going to be OK. At some point during the visit, however, I make sure they hear from me something they may have already intuited: the First Lesson of Parenthood is "You're not in control."

For any attentive person this side of the grave, the First Lesson of Parenthood (the acronym for which is, fittingly enough, FLOP) should come as no surprise, but the modern—and, in many ways, distinctively American—mythologies of autonomy and self-creation obscure the obvious. Contrary to glib assurances that we can make things come out right in the end, the bumper sticker says, "Shit Happens." Wishing things otherwise won't prevent disaster. With disaster comes grief, the ingredients of which are love, loss, and memory, and the greatest of these is love. No matter how much Buddhist detachment or Osler's stoic dispassion one cultivates, love—especially familial love—is grief's midwife. "Somehow one's dreadfully vulnerable through those one loves," wrote the novelist and physicist, C. P. Snow.[1] I know that to be true, know it far better than many of my convictions. I know it from close observation and personal grief.

I was a pediatrician before I was a father. I cared for other people's children before being graced with my own. When Will—our first—was born, I held his scrawny six pounds, eight ounces in one arm, looked into those blinking, bluish-gray eyes with expanding wonder, and whispered over and again, "You're my little baby boy." I was in love and newly vulnerable.

In adding the title "father" to my pediatrician's resume, the things that didn't change surprised me as much as what did. A new vulnerability didn't alter my approach to painful procedures like spinal taps and IVs.

1. Snow, *The Masters*, 6.

Pediatric training made clear when and why such things—however un-pleasant—must be done. Loving my children doesn't alter that. If anything, parenthood strengthened my sense that what tools I have should be used when necessary.

But Will's birth placed child illness and suffering in a new, disturbing context. Parental distress over a child in pain was no longer an abstraction. When Will was in the throes of colic, I learned what it was like to walk the house with a baby who will not be consoled. When my Peter awoke with a fever, I learned what fears uncertainty conjures. And, just as desire is often sweeter than possession, uncertainty is often worse than knowing what we call "the worst." A diagnosis at least names the enemy.

With a child of my own, dependent on his parents for nearly every-thing, what had once been throwaway lines like "the fragility of life" lodged in my throat. It wasn't what I had to do to a sick infant that bothered me, but the threat illness posed to my child. This is precisely where a dose of Osler's detachment is helpful: dwell too much on emotional identification, and the good a doctor might do slips away like sand through a crack in the floor.

I promised myself never to play pediatrician for my own children, knowing what mistakes befall those who confuse roles. For years, I declined even the children of friends as patients, afraid the slightest blurring of lines could render me stupider than usual. In time, though, I learned to negotiate lesser forms of role confusion, as my children and their many quirks weaned me from much professional dogmatism. I still recited standard recommen-dations for feeding, sleep, and discipline, but added, when appropriate, my hard-won awareness that children rarely follow the manuals, that "normal" is a fluid term and "best" an ideal rarely achieved. One of the smartest physi-cians I know regularly lectures her residents on child behavior modification techniques. She knows the professional recommendations to the letter, and guarantees her listeners that if a parent does "X" properly and consistently, the child will—as night follows day—do "Y." Her confidence is charming, but until and unless she has children of her own, I find her recommenda-tions unpersuasive.

* * * *

In times of uncertainty, simple tasks become blessings, distracting an obses-sive mind if not truly comforting it. Deciding aloud to take Peter to the hospital filled Jill and me with purpose. Jill called Katie, our neighbor, to watch Will while we tended to Peter's illness. Will was the only person in our house who had slept through the night, and he would soon be ready for an active day. Playing with Katie's kids might corral his enthusiasm while we dealt with Peter's medical issues. I phoned Steve, the pediatrician on call, who told us to meet him in the Emergency Department in fifteen minutes. It took all of five minutes to walk from our house to the hospital, more than enough time to gather our things, drop Will off at Katie's, and carry Peter to the ED.

The late November morning was brisk, and we walked with determination down the street and into the main ED entrance. Jill carried Peter in her arms, wrapped in a blanket. The ED nurse took Peter's temperature when we arrived. 100.8: better, but still a fever for someone Peter's age. Steve met us in the exam room. He asked us standard questions: what happened and when, and what we'd done for Peter so far. Then, after doing a quick exam, including listening to Peter's chest and peering in his ears and throat, Steve turned to us and said, "Well, I think you know what I have to do next."

We did. At least I did. Jill knew some of what was coming, too, though not to the same detail as I. Steve asked us if we wanted to step out while he collected specimens of blood, urine, and spinal fluid. I'd performed LPs ("lumbar punctures"—doctor-speak for spinal taps) on babies while a parent watched and knew the unspoken pressure an audience puts on the doctor, so I turned to Jill and said, "Let's go."

With a divided sense that we were abandoning our child and doing precisely what he most needed, we left the room. We stayed indoors, out of the cold morning air, and circuited the hospital hallways, past the lab and medical records to the front entrance, down the long hallway past the dental, family medicine, and pediatric clinics, then by the inpatient units at the far end before turning back toward the ED. The hospital was deserted so early on Thanksgiving Day. The waiting rooms were empty and the lights dimmed. Jill and I made small talk as we made our rounds once, twice, three times. We walked slowly, mostly arm in arm, trying not to think too much about the one person who most concerned us, while Peter, infant though he was, trudged alongside—or rather, between us—an invisible third party on our silent march.

When, at last, we heard our names paged overhead, calling us back to the ED, we sped there directly. Steve met us outside the exam room and reassured as all had gone well. Peter was on the bed asleep, the ordeal of the spinal tap having strangely calmed him, as I'd seen with so many other infants. He had a cotton ball taped to the back of a hand where blood had been drawn, a band aid low in his back where the spinal needle had entered, and an IV in one arm. Jill and I carried him to the hospital room where he would spend the next two days, down the far hallway of the pediatric unit, past the room where Alice had died, all the way to the end, where the nurses had prepared the room.

We waited awhile until Steve came by to tell us initial results from the blood, urine, and spinal fluid. All reassuringly suggested a viral illness. This was good news, but not enough information to send us home. Proof lay in the cultures, and we'd wait until Saturday morning to have results final enough for discharge. There was nothing to do until then but watch and wait while Peter received antibiotics through his IV—with a febrile baby, one assumes a bacterial infection until proven otherwise—and comfort our son as best we could.

Jill and I discussed dividing the tasks ahead. Will was at Katie's and could stay several more hours, though Katie and her husband, Joe, had Thanksgiving plans themselves later on. We'd have to relieve them sometime. For now, however, we both needed sleep. Jill had no intention of leaving Peter's side and told me to fetch some of her things from home. After that, she said, I should go back home, and we'd both try to get some rest. It was a task—a welcome one—and I did as I was told.

* * * *

If the First Lesson of Parenthood—"You're not in control"—were simply an intellectual achievement, it could be learned and used as a universal formula, like Newton's Second Law of Motion, where force always equals mass times acceleration. Even in a world of friction, guesstimates, and chaos, Newton's Second Law should be as simple as plugging in the values and doing the math. But the First Lesson of Parenthood is neither an intellectual nor a single achievement. It's too large a blow to the ego for most to master readily. Those who imagine they've thoroughly learned the First Lesson will be forced to learn it all over again.

I learned it again when Will, then three years old, made the softest of splashes as he fell over the side of a beached raft into the swift water of the San Juan River. That Jill heard the sound in a moment of shared parental inattention is one more piece of evidence that mothers, not fathers, are the key to child survival. Jill dropped what she was holding, plunged blindly into the water, and fished our son out—losing her glasses in the process—before I knew what had happened.

Jill and I learned it again when Peter came home from preschool complaining that his elbow hurt. At the time, it wasn't enough to slow him down, but over several hours the elbow grew increasingly swollen and tender. Once more, we found ourselves in an Emergency Room, and when the orthopedic resident drew pus from Peter's elbow in a syringe, I knew again where we were headed—the operating room, on overnight stay (or more), and a long course of antibiotics. I also caught myself listing potential complications—some minor, others terrifying—along the way to recovery. I retreated to my fortress of knowledge, even as the walls settled unevenly into bogs of fear and anxiety.

Many parents adapt, at least initially, to the First Lesson by worrying, as if compulsive thought might alter reality. Like a caged panther, the mind circles, searching for a gap in the iron bars. Some were accomplished worriers before becoming parents, but the vulnerability accompanying a new child can unhinge the calmest soul. In time, parenthood may lead beyond worry to acceptance of what little one can control, to take the rest of life as it comes: as a given, perhaps even as a gift. It doesn't make parenting any easier, nor does it relieve the feeling that we're making this up as we go along, since we are, in fact, making it up as we go along. As children grow older, parenting becomes a game of whack-a-mole: with each new crisis beaten down, another pops up, near-adults devising new and ingenious ways to complicate their lives and ours. As the Assistant Dean of the medical school said, "It doesn't get any better; it just gets different."

With age, I've come to see parenthood as a lens through which to glimpse my powerlessness. It's always been there, like a distant planet circling the sun, but it takes a powerful telescope to spy it. Life is generously supplied with similar lenses: unrequited love, natural disasters, death. Each encounter, however indirect or brief, refocuses my wandering attention on some personal vulnerability I can't escape without shedding—as I have no wish to do—my body and my affections. As theologian Miroslav Volf says, "vulnerability is the essential condition of human life. No vulnerability, no human life."[2]

* * * *

From her chair alongside Peter's hospital crib, Jill issued marching orders. I walked home, gathered necessaries—a change of clothes, toiletries, snacks, fruit, a can of sparkling water, some papers from work, and a book for Jill to read if time and worry permitted—put them in a tote bag, and carried them back to the hospital. Jill had Peter to the breast when I arrived, our son as fussy as ever.

"Can I get you anything else?" I asked, setting her things on the window ledge. "Should I stay?"

2. Volf, Sarah Smith Memorial Conference, Welcoming Remarks.

"No and no," Jill said. "He'll fall asleep again soon and then I'll sleep, too. You go, get some rest, and then pick up Will from Katie's."

And so I went home and slept—neither well nor long, but enough to clear some of the world-blurring fatigue from my eyes. I made myself a sandwich, then walked to Katie's. Will and Meghan, Katie's oldest daughter, were watching a video. Katie was in the kitchen, cleaning up.

"Oh, you're here," Katie said. "I thought you'd stay at the hospital or sleep at home."

"I figured you needed a break from Will," I said.

"As you can see," she said, pointing toward the television with her chin and lip in the Navajo way, "they're doing fine. Will can stay all day."

"Don't you have Thanksgiving plans?" I asked.

"We're just going over to Sharon's and Tony's. You should come, too." Sharon and Tony were our next-door neighbors. It sounded like the usual Tuba City gathering, where more are always welcome. Rather than answering Katie immediately, I pondered how we might get Jill and me to Sharon's together.

Seeing my indecision, Katie added, "I'm assuming you've cancelled the rest of your weekend plans." She knew Jill and I had made reservations for a room outside Zion National Park. We'd planned to drive there with the boys on Friday and stay two nights. We hadn't told many people about the trip, but clearly Jill had spoken to Katie about it. One person we'd been careful not to tell was our Hopi baby sitter, Edna. Edna lived in Moencopi, a Hopi village across the highway from Tuba City, and she'd been our babysitter since Will was born. There were two reasons we'd kept Edna in the dark about our plans for the long weekend. The first was that we'd planned to do a very Navajo thing while in Zion, and Jill didn't know what Edna would make of it. The Navajo tradition is to bury a baby's placenta where the family wishes the child to be rooted. For a Navajo boy, that might be in the sheep corral; for a girl, under grandmother's loom. The child then has a bodily link to a traditional place and practice. When Will was born, we didn't keep the placenta, but we saved the stump of his umbilical cord when it fell off and buried it in a particularly lovely spot in Zion National Park. We intended to do the same for Peter, symbolically rooting them both in a part of the world Jill and I loved. Edna had been particularly generous with her Hopi tradition regarding the boys, giving them both Hopi names and making sure there were presents for them at *Powamu*, the Hopi Bean Dance held in the lower village in early February. Edna wasn't necessarily opposed to us doing Navajo things. She had no complaints when we had a party to celebrate Will's first laugh, an occasion of great community significance for the Navajo. On the other hand, Edna said and did things to make clear she knew far more about children in general—and ours in particular—than Jill or me. Having raised six kids of her own, that was no doubt true in many ways, but Jill often felt Edna was second-guessing her.

We never asked Edna about her feelings on burying cord stumps. I have no doubt, however, that she would have scolded us for taking Peter out of house that weekend. Traditional Hopis keep newborns indoors for nearly three weeks after birth. On the twentieth day, the family gathers for a party at which each relative gives the child a name. Edna didn't expect us to do that with Peter—we certainly hadn't done it with Will—but we knew from experience that Edna forever worried about "her baby" being outside or getting cold, both of which she saw as a sure path to sickness. That Jill and I were physicians made no difference. Edna knew for certain what caused illness in children and shared her medical opinions freely. Even though we planned to do very little outside the cabin in Utah, I wondered myself whether it was still too early to take Peter, that he'd get sick from a virus caught on our excursion. As it turned out, Peter got sick without ever leaving home.

I was rehearsing all this in my mind as soon as Katie asked about cancelling our plans and she took note of my long silence: "I mean, I assume you're not going to Utah while Peter's in the hospital."

"No. Of course we're not going."

"Either way, you should come to Sharon's tonight." Which is what I ended up doing, having spent the day following the advice of women who, as usual, knew better than I what to do in troubled times.

* * * *

I love my father and still grieve a decade after his death. His absence is heaviest when I ache with love for my own children and question. I needn't idealize my father beyond what he was in life. His almost-hidden struggle with depression and self-doubt renders his person that much more familiar to me, yet he loved us—and my mother most of all—with the ferocity of a glowing coal, shedding constant light and more warmth than flame. I hope to live according to his example.

Becoming a father means welcoming an unknown, dependent person who never consented to the deal, who's full of demands, and who learns the location of your many faults and hot buttons. Here again, the First Lesson of Parenthood applies: I may strive to be open, nurturing, and affirming to my children but can't control how things turn out. I can't even know if I've passed the midterms, uncertain as I am how to measure my efforts. But in my best days, I share with the title character in Wendell Berry's novel, *Jayber Crow,* the conviction that the name, "father," implies a fraught tangle of realities: "the love, the compassion, the taking offense, the disappointment, the anger, the bearing of wounds, the weeping of tears, the forgiveness . . ."[3]

* * * *

The remainder of Thanksgiving Day filled with busywork, tasks that kept my mind sufficiently occupied to muzzle its fears. In between chores, I checked in with Jill, who refused to leave Peter's side and said she had all she needed for now. Will, for whom a younger brother was still a novelty, asked to see Peter, but decided he'd rather play with Meghan and Kevin, another neighbor down the street, when I told him the hospital didn't let three year-olds visit sick children. Neighbors inquired after Peter and asked what I was doing for dinner that night. Feeling vulnerable and in no mood to talk long, I answered in short statements of fact: "He's doing well. It's probably a virus. The cultures will tell. We're eating at Sharon and Tony's."

Though I found the prospect of answering yet more questions at a party unappealing, I looked forward to Thanksgiving dinner, which would be the standard neighborhood potluck, everyone bringing something. Potlucks were Tuba City's moveable feasts, forever familiar and new. Most of the hospital professionals—doctors, nurses, and therapists—lived in modular government townhouses. The only differences were the number of bedrooms and whether the dining area and kitchen stood to the left or right of the living room. We otherwise knew what to expect—save the food, which depended on who was coming and how much time they had to prepare.

During a visit to the hospital late that afternoon, Jill and I made plans for the evening. Will and I would go to Sharon and Tony's. Jill would join us when she could get Peter to sleep. Afterward, she would spend the night with Peter in the hospital while I stayed home with Will. I say *we* were making these plans, but I mostly took notes. My talents include theory and grand ideas. Jill's are more practical. With matters so topsy-turvy, I valued direction over agency. If Jill needed anything, I could find it when she came to dinner. I leaned over to kiss her, placed another kiss on the sweaty forehead of my son, and headed home.

Sharon and Tony lived next door to us. A cottonwood tree rooted on their side of the fence spread widely, shading both homes. As I walked to their door to join the Thanksgiving Day dinner, the sun sank below the roofline on the far side of the house row. Inside was the familiar hospital

3. Berry, *Jayber Crow,* 251.

gathering, the group who had become our surrogate extended family on the Reservation. Faces turned my way, registering a mixture of welcome and compassion. I grinned with resolute cheeriness and stepped further in. Will was in the corner, playing with Jenny, Sharon and Tony's daughter. What had been a day from hell for Jill and me had turned into a rotating play date for our firstborn, another gift from the neighborhood's mothers. The kids were easier to look at than my colleagues and friends, whose glances of empathy already felt oppressive, no matter how well-intentioned. Was this how I looked to the parents of my sick patients?

Around the corner, a feast covered the dining table, from steaming turkey meat to a bowl of blue corn mush. I realized I'd forgotten to bring something to add. I turned to Sharon and sheepishly apologized for arriving empty handed.

"Nonsense," she said, "You had better things to do, and there's no way we'll finish all this," pointing to the table and the stacked kitchen beyond. I appreciated her kindness, though like many Anglo medical profession-als, I learned from Navajo or Hopi babysitters the prime directive of Native hospitality: always bring something.

There was nothing to do now, however, and for the first time in hours, I was hungry. I filled my plate. Jill arrived soon thereafter. She was hungry, too, but equally desperate to talk with someone other than a nurse about her day. I gladly let her answer everyone's questions about Peter while I stood at her side. Like me, she'd made up for lost sleep in brief snatches, and her eyes spoke of worry and fatigue, but I was happy to be with someone to whom I didn't have to explain things. There's a good reason parents gener-ally come in twos.

We didn't stay long that evening. I made my rounds of thank yous and good nights and gathered Will to go home while Jill made some last minute conversations with friends. It was good to see her animated, even in her weariness. Will came reluctantly, his long and nearly perfect day over at last. The three of us made the short walk to our house and prepared for the night. Jill brushed her teeth, found an extra blanket and a change of clothes, and stopped at the front door before walking back to the hospital. We held each other quietly enough to hear one another's breathing, a reassurance I'd miss that night in my otherwise empty bed. I told her I'd be by early next morning. Then she headed out the door.

"Come on, Will," I called. "We both need to get to bed."

I arose early from a welcome night of uninterrupted sleep, made a pot of coffee, and called the pediatric unit at the hospital. The nurses brought Jill to the phone, and she said, with a yawn, that her night, too, had gone well. Peter slept and apparently felt better. He'd just nursed and was once again asleep.

"How about we switch places?" I said. "You come home to clean up, rest a little, and be with Will, and I sit with Peter for a few hours."

"Sounds great," Jill said, and we did just that, meeting at the door minutes later, repeating last night's goodbye with roles exchanged. My morning walk to the hospital was less ominous than it had been only the day before, the November sun just as bright but noticeably warmer. A car engine sputtered in the distance. Dry leaves stirred in the breeze. Except for the very few who'd driven away long before daybreak to shop in Flagstaff, the town slept late the day after Thanksgiving.

It was equally quiet in the hospital. A nurse held a phone to her ear at the nurses' station, looking more like she was on hold than intently listening. Another nurse moved down the opposite hallway from Peter's room. Peter himself was still asleep, his chest rising and falling easily, his hair neatly combed. The Navajo and Hopi nurses were taken by this rarity—an Anglo baby born with a full head of black hair—and enjoyed keeping it neat.

Steve poked his head in the door and said, "He's doing great. No fever overnight and the cultures are still negative."

"Thanks," I said, with an unforced smile. If the cultures remained negative—that is, with no bacterial growth detected—through tomorrow morning, forty-eight hours after they'd been drawn, we could go home, reasonably sure this had been no more than virus. From now until then, there was little more to do than wait. With the First Lesson of Parenthood comes equally unwelcome tutelage in the practice of patience. Only hours stood between Peter and hospital discharge—about twenty-three just then—and puttering, pacing, and worrying wouldn't speed things up. Later improvements in lab detection have since shortened the process, but bacteria can be rushed only so much.

Peter made up for lost sleep. I sat in a chair and looked out the window at the parking lot and the town beyond. Is this what mothers and fathers did while I wrote medical orders on their children or looked at X rays? I picked up a book and tried to read, but found myself skimming pages without retaining a word. In the end, I took the hint from my son, closed my eyes, and attended to the rise and fall of my chest, thinking of as little as possible, quieting as best I could the chaos of my mind.

Before Peter woke up, Jill returned, looking better rested if not fully refreshed. "Will's at Katy's again this morning," she said. "We owe them big."

"Yes," I said. "We do."

Jill and I sat together, catching up on each other's past day. We talked through shared exhaustion, powerless over our most urgent, shared concern.

I wondered how parents of chronically ill children keep their wits while love and fear tug in opposite directions. After little more than a day, we were already fraying. For most, I suppose, the answer is fairly simple: find a way to go on. I admire those who do, but it's admiration without envy. For young parents like us, who knew too much about what can go wrong in a hospital, our crash course couldn't end soon enough.

The rest of Friday passed uneventfully. Peter was clearly on the mend, feeding vigorously and looking, while awake, happier than his parents. Jill and I traded places throughout the day. Will asked about Peter, and appeared satisfied his brother would likely come home tomorrow.

Sleep, that welcome healer of hurts, came readily to all that night, and the following morning passed as expected. All cultures were negative, Steve wrote discharge orders, and our nurse removed Peter's IV and patient wristband. We were going home.

It felt excessive to use the car—a four wheel drive Isuzu Trooper we bought to travel reservation back roads and dirt trails—for a route I usually walked, but we'd accumulated more items over the course of two days than we could carry in one trip. We were also anxious to shield Peter from the November chill. Though I knew—contrary to Edna's warnings—that viruses, not temperature, caused colds, I was now the parent of a vulnerable child. More accurately, I was vulnerable through my child. If affections undermined reason, so be it. We drove to our house on East Elm Circle—a loop conspicuously lacking elm trees—and reconstituted our young family of four under one roof.

Will thrilled to see Peter again, speaking to him in high-pitched, reassuring tones about the fun they would soon share. But novelty soon lost its shine, and he suggested we watch a video while Jill put Peter to bed. I didn't resist. We had no grand plan other than to be together. The remainder of the day unfolded with little surprise, not through some reassertion of control, but because none of us attempted or expected much.

Over a dinner of reheated leftovers that evening, Jill and I discussed what to do with Peter's cord stump, which we had planned to bury in Zion National Park. Though neither of us were Native and had no patience for Wannabes—Anglo pretenders who commandeer Native practices, torn from any cultural context, for personal consumption—the simple ritual of rooting our child to a familiar place of great beauty tugged at our hearts.

"I'd still like to do something with it, even if Zion's too long of a drive for a one-day trip," Jill said.

"How about the Grand Canyon?" I suggested.

"Even with a baby, the South Rim would be an easy afternoon trip," Jill said.

I pulled out a National Park Service map and looked for likely spots. If Jill or I had our druthers, we'd rather be on the North Rim, where only 10 percent of the park's visitors go, but it was already closed for the winter, gathering snowpack as we spoke. I suggested a trailhead on the South Rim that Jill and I had set out from on hikes to the river, a respectful distance from the bustle of Grand Canyon Village. The place had good memories for us both, and we agreed to drive there the following afternoon.

By Sunday morning, Peter's illness was only an unsettling memory. Jill, unwilling to risk too much exposure for our young son, stayed home with both boys while I went to St. Jude's for Mass, where Anglo and Navajo friends asked how Peter was doing, what they could do for us, and when we planned to baptize him. For once, I welcomed the questions, genuinely grateful for simple gestures of community. Many well-wishers, more familiar with illness and uncertainty than I, passed over their own experiences in silence, save to acknowledge that they, too, understood the frightening powerlessness at the heart of parenthood. The corollary to the First Law of Parenthood, I began to grasp, is the Declaration of Interdependence: "We're in this together."

I drove home and walked in the front door. Will poked his head around the corner and grinned with mischief. "Can you smell our surprise?" he said.

I sniffed. "Smells like you made something good for us to eat."

"Mom and I made pancakes!" Will shouted, his face bursting with excitement and pride, as if he'd scaled a mountain.

"I can't wait to taste them," I said, "I'm hungry."

"Good," Will said, his blonde hair bounced as he quivered, "We made lots."

"Take your seats at the table," Jill called from the kitchen, and Will and I did.

Jill brought the last items to the table in one hand, holding Peter to her shoulder with the other. I offered to take him, but Jill insisted, "We just nursed and he's nearly asleep." And so we ate.

Hot pancakes with butter and real maple syrup, glasses of pulpy orange juice, and mugs of coffee with cream felt more a family feast than the rushed affair Thanksgiving dinner had been. The latter had been an act of gracious hospitality for which we were grateful, but this unhurried family meal, made by those I loved, was far more precious. We lingered at our places, Peter nodding off to sleep, Will telling us about his past two days, Jill and I sharing the pleasure of our sons' company.

Afterward, Will and Jill cleared the table while I washed the dishes. We bundled up the boys—it was chillier than any of the past three days—and gathered the baby necessaries in a bag. We loaded the Trooper, Peter in his car seat and Will in his booster, and set off for the South Rim.

We drove through landscape that once had seemed to us forbidding, desolate as an asteroid. If, as Anglos, we never truly become native to this place, we nonetheless come to call it home, learning the names of places, adopting its habits, respecting its wildness and power. We passed treeless red rocks near Moenave, the crudely painted sign pointing the way to real dinosaur tracks, the black magmatic dike of an ancient volcano, the layered, rainbow mudstones of the Chinle formation with its clusters of petrified logs: evidence of forces and timescales that dwarfed us. We turned south at the intersection with Route 89, past Shadow Mountain, the dry riverbed of the Little Colorado, and the trading post at Cameron. There were houses and hogans, some abandoned. We couldn't see the interiors: how many people slept in single rooms, the drafty chinks under doors and windows. We didn't see the lives already lost: infants who didn't make it to the hospital in time, children crushed under the wheels of a pickup, men and women whose hidden wounds compelled them to drink alcohol from cans of hair spray before they died. Nor could we see the abandoned wells contaminated with uranium from the mining boom.

From Cameron, we turned west toward the looming ridge of Grey Mountain, our route paralleling the dark, undulating gash of the Little Colorado Canyon until we ascended the Coconino Plateau. As we climbed, we passed from desert scrub through stands of Juniper and Pinyon, and finally to thick forests of Ponderosa Pine, a progression determined by altitude, temperature, and rainfall with more precision than humans could hope for. Plants and animals live where they survive. Doing otherwise courts death. The desert is an unforgiving landscape where the necessity of accepting what can't change grows more pressing, the folly of human designs more apparent.

From his seat in the back, Will asked for music. Jill slipped in a tape of songs about the Grand Canyon, and Will sang along, first at full voice, then more softly, until the drone of the car lulled him to sleep. Peter napped much of the drive. For a long while, Jill and I said almost nothing, both of us seasoning thoughts of the past days with images of the land we called home. At last, Jill broke the silence: "Being a parent is scary."

"Yes, it is," I agreed, thinking Jill had finished her thought.

"The thing is," she continued, "as a mom, I want to protect my kids. You can say nasty things about me all day long, but you threaten my kids and I become the Momma Bear defending her cubs. I'm ready to rip out somebody's lungs. But what if its not a person threatening your child? What if it's a big rock, or ice on the road, or germs? What do I do then? How can I protect my babies?"

"I don't know, Jill. I don't know."

For us, of course, no one had died. No one had been permanently injured. We had had a brief, minor scare. That's all. I'd seen much worse as a doctor, seen Brian and Alice die, all my efforts to save them useless. I needed no reminders, having spent much of my professional time worrying about what could go wrong with children under my care. It's different when the child you worry about is your own. Context matters, and few contexts prove more powerful than love.

We arrived at the point where we planned to bury Peter's cord. I pulled the Trooper as close as I could before cutting the ignition. I noted with approval that we were alone at the chilly overlook. We would have the place to ourselves, with no one to ask what we were doing, digging a hole in a National Park.

"Well," I said, "shall we all get out?"

"No," Jill said, "I'm not taking Peter out in this cold."

Will was still asleep, undisturbed by the car coming to a halt.

"You go ahead," Jill said, "I'll watch from here."

I picked up the envelope in which we'd placed Peter's cord stump, opened the driver's door, and stepped outside, zipping my parka up to my neck against the chill. The ground was snowless. That, I knew, would change in the next few weeks. I walked to a limestone outcropping pocked with holes and shallow depressions and looked out into the canyon, its layers of colored rock marked in uneven steps. The river still carving the canyon lay hidden at its center, shielded from view by the sudden, deep slope of the inner gorge. I listened for ravens, but only heard wind in the pines. Then came the chirp of a bird—a chickadee, I thought—in the trees nearby. To my right, a nuthatch scaled headfirst down a roughened trunk, pecking now and then for insects. It was an island of tenacious life, a beachhead in a stony sea of erosion and loss.

The soil around me—where there was any—gathered in shallow basins and crevices in the limestone surface. I found a spot, deeper than most, and dug with my hands, having forgotten a trowel. I turned from the small hole to open the envelope. Inside, wrapped in a paper towel, was an inch-long piece of dry flesh looking like a piece of jerky. To me it was beautiful, if only because it had come into the world with my son, fed by his blood and marked with his DNA.

I placed it at the bottom of the hole and paused for a moment to whisper a word of thanks before covering it with dirt, then tamped the ground flat with the sole of my shoe. I looked around me once more, fixing the place in my memory so I could find it again.

"Did it go OK?" Jill asked as I climbed behind the wheel.

"Yes," I said. "I'm glad we chose here. It's a gorgeous place."

"I'm glad, too," Jill said. "No matter what Peter does or doesn't do, no matter what happens to him, there will always be a bit of him here."

"Yes," I said. I reached to turn the key. "No matter what happens."

Chapter Five

Reading the Body

Tuba City, Navajo Nation

HENRY WAS IN PAIN. It didn't take a doctor to diagnose that from the way he limped behind the clinic nurse. Marie, the short Hopi LPN, pattered toward my exam room at the end of the hallway as Henry fell farther behind, bent stiffly forward at the waist, his right hand pressed discreetly to his belly. When I entered the room myself, chart in hand, Henry leaned against the exam table, slump-shouldered and anxious.

Henry was no talker. Like most Navajo boys, he made little of his discomfort, and spoke with frustrating vagueness about what may have been a fever and what sounded like sudden loss of appetite. Henry couldn't remember if he'd vomited or when he last took pain medicine. This, at least, was certain: he wasn't about to tell me his diagnosis, at least not directly.

Where does one start in such a case? I like to imagine I'm trained to think analytically, dissecting the body's secrets with scalpels of science. Henry presented a challenge, more so than the steady parade of diarrhea, stuffy noses, and infected ears making up the bulk of a pediatrician's day. I asked him to sit on the table. He slowly pushed himself upward, his hands pressed against the table's edge, in a conspicuous effort not to move faster than he had to.

"This is hurting you a lot," I said.

"No," he said, the vowel cut short like a root sliced through with a spade.

I began my exam, trusting Henry's body to tell me what he wouldn't or couldn't, moving quickly over the head, eyes, ears, throat, and neck, lingering a moment over chest and heart before moving on to the belly.

I asked him to lie down. Slowly, carefully, he lowered his back and head to the white paper crinkling on the cushioned table. I offered help, but he refused. He lay still at last, eyeing me carefully for any sudden, potentially painful move. And just then, before I lifted his shirt to see his abdomen, I remembered what I was doing.

The examination of a patient's abdomen, like any part of the physical exam, is a skill learned early in medical education, a habitual practice the physician adopts in becoming a healer. I wince at my younger self's awkward entry into the long line of clinicians, under the eye of mentors kind enough not to comment on my quavering voice or my trembling hands, half-hidden in the sleeves of a spotless white coat. Medicine—till then mostly theoretical—became terrifyingly real, with living bodies healed or harmed by my touch. My mind, used to piloting the ship, was suddenly at sea without a compass. I knew the names of the classic texts, though I'd barely skimmed Cope's *Early Diagnosis of the Acute Abdomen*. And I was blessed with a voracious memory—invaluable in this profession—gobbling up lists, sequences and a word-lover's treasure of medical eponyms: Murphy's sign, McBurney's point, Crohn disease. But the real learning began bedside, apprenticed to a master, the experienced physician demonstrating: "This is how we examine. Do this." And I did. Many, many times. The old saw in medical teaching is: "See one, do one, teach one." It's nearly true. More accurately, it's: "See one, do hundreds, teach, and learn it again."

Henry's pain dwelled in his belly, I was sure. To lure it into the open, I laid traps I learned in medical school, dividing the abdominal exam into the traditional four parts, performed in standard order: observation, auscultation, percussion, and palpation. I must remain conscious of the organs beneath the visible flesh, the connectedness of the belly to what lies above and below, and Henry's response to my every move. The abdomen can't be separated from the patient the way a mechanic services a car's gas pump by first removing it.

Observation. I rubbed my hands to warm them and stood at Henry's right side, his head to my left. My eyes traced the contour of his belly—the long curve of another Navajo boy too fond of Taco Bell, Coca Cola, and fry bread made with lard. The dome curved symmetrically, unscarred by surgery, undistorted by whatever trouble lay underneath. I watched it rise and fall with each breath. Henry was subtly splinting, keeping his right side still to limit pain caused by movement. I was getting somewhere.

Henry watched me carefully, his eyes intent on my hands, not my face. He feared my touch. This hurt far more than he let on. Before I set my hand to his skin, I warmed the diaphragm of my stethoscope in my palms and turned my attention from sight to sound.

Auscultation. I lightly touched the stethoscope to the upper left quadrant of his belly, as far from where I guessed he hurt as I could go. I slowly moved the diaphragm down his left flank, pausing to listen for the squeaks and gurgles of healthy digestion. What I heard instead were rare, distant, high-pitched tones, like the call of a reclusive bird. Now moving down his right side, I listened first, then pressed the diaphragm slightly deeper, using my stethoscope, that elegant invention of Rene Theophile Hyacinthe Laennec. Laennec was a nineteenth-century French physician too sensitive and polite to press his ear to the chest of a portly young woman with heart disease. He solved the problem by making a hollow cylinder, putting one end to the patient's chest and placing his ear on the other end. Stethoscopes look very different now, but his inventive response to a troubled sense of propriety revolutionized the art of physical diagnosis, enhancing the ear's role. In examining Henry, however, I was using the eye as much as the ear, carefully observing his response to the pressure of my stethoscope on his belly, watching for clues to separate histrionics from true pain. Henry flinched. No doubt here. His right lower quadrant was tender. Possible appendicitis?

Percussion. After seeing Henry's reaction to light pressure, I didn't want to cause more discomfort than necessary. I'd normally sound out the length and breadth of his belly next, my left hand flat against the skin, striking my left middle finger with the tip of the right, flipping the right hand downward with the hinged wrist of a catcher tossing out a runner at second. With the ear of a vintner inspecting wine barrels, I'd listen for the dullness within, noting where this gives way to the drum-like resonance of air-filled cavities. Faced with a tender abdomen, though, I had to be gentle. As I sounded his liver, high on his belly's right side, his eyes began to tear. I apologized and stopped.

Palpation. Laying my left hand flat high on the right side of Henry's belly, I slowly pressed the fingers of my right hand just behind the nails of my left. To palpate with just one hand risks missing the subtler aspects of the exam. The sensitive pads of the fingers discover more than the fingertips. I moved slowly over his belly, letting Henry anticipate my progress, saving the right lower quadrant for last. Beginning with light pressure, I proceeded to deeper interrogation, watching for rebound tenderness—increased pain with sudden removal of the palpating hand—a sign of peritonitis, inflam-mation of the abdominal lining. Once again, he hurt most on his right lower side, though he didn't appear to hurt more on rebound. If his appendix was inflamed, perhaps it had not yet ruptured.

I now had valuable information, having read in Henry's body what he did not tell me in words. I ordered blood work and X rays of his abdomen and chest—I'd been fooled before into diagnosing appendicitis when the real problem was pneumonia—but my real task was notifying the surgeons. I'd leave the rectal exam to them—an essential diagnostic maneuver, but one I deferred, knowing the surgeons would repeat it even if I'd already done one. I chose not to hurt my patient more than necessary.

I thanked Henry for his cooperation, told him what I was worried about and that I had to make some calls, and stepped out of the room. Later that evening, I stopped by Henry's room on the pediatric unit. He slept, his chest rising and falling in slow cadence. An IV snaked to his arm. I didn't lift the sheet to inspect the bandage. Bruce, one of the surgeons, told me what I wanted to know: Henry's appendix, grossly inflamed and recently ruptured, was already on its way to the pathologist. The surgery went smoothly.

"Too bad we didn't get it before it burst," Bruce said. "Boys here tough these things out."

I agreed. Maybe if Henry had come in earlier. But we'd done what we had to with what we were given. Henry would do fine.

I don't remember the note I wrote in Henry's chart that day in pediatric clinic, but I know what form it took. The medical note, a genre so conven-tional it rarely rises above cliché, starts with a chief complaint—ideally in the patient's words—followed by a brief introductory exposition. In Henry's case, this probably went something like "This twelve year old boy presents with a three day history of nausea, low grade fever and abdominal pain." The rest of the history—Henry's story as I heard and interpreted it—followed in standard sequence: present illness, past medical history, family history, so-cial history, and review of systems. Physical exam came next, starting with weight and vital signs—temperature, respirations, pulse and blood pres-sure—and moving from head to toe, with the abdominal exam coming, in the natural order of things, between chest and genitals. Each stanza has an internal order, summing the data of my senses, what I had seen, heard, and felt of Henry's body. If the labs and X rays were available before I finished my note, the results appeared farther down the page. Last, an assessment—probable appendicitis—and plan—surgery consulted, patient to go to OR today. The aim of such scribbling is to move the patient's story toward an acceptable denouement: pain relief, mind relief, or something like it.

That's how doctors tell stories. It's often how we find the story in the first place, the plot taking first form in the telling. My colleagues and I still share puzzling cases by presenting them, in standard fashion, to one another. The practice itself clarifies, assembling pieces in a verbal arrow flying, we trust, toward a conclusion. We may learn, in time, how wrong our first telling was. New information twists the narrative arc into strange shapes. Important details, glossed over in a hasty first reading, come to light. Doctors misapprehend, discover things only in hindsight, make mistakes. We hope none of them are fatal, that crucial information—like the fluid around Brian's heart—isn't hidden from us, doesn't require an autopsy to be discovered. We hope to learn from our missed chances with as little harm to others as possible. We hope that our patients as well as our stories improve with experience.

But as long as humans are mortal, there is only one true end to every story. One final diagnosis fits all. For all the promises of Enlightenment dreamers and transhumanist tinkerers, medical science has managed only to defer death, not master it. Doctors tell medical stories in part to control what little we can. Modern medicine, like politics, is an art of the possible. We narrate our patients to a place where our tools make a difference, a verbal diversion from the vast fields of futility. Before we begin, before we speak or write a word of any patient's story, mortality is already drawing its closed border, defining the territory in which a life's drama plays out. Doctors go astray if we forget that.

This is the narrative form I entered, a tradition handed to me by masters, and which I hope to hand on, in turn, to others. It is, I tell my students as they present their patients, a window into habits of thought. History and physical narrate not only the patient, but the examiner as well: how we approach our patients, what we attend to, what we apprehend.

It's also a way of reading. I remember Howard Nemerov's graduate student, the one who looked up from the page they were studying together to announce, "I see what reading is. It's putting together what you've got with what it says." It works for medicine, too. Formed by years of training and the reading of many bodies, physicians put what they've got with what they find, intuiting the shape of health or disease from signs written in flesh. To read well is to have read often, and medicine's shiny new tools—scans, informatics and Internet searches—while immensely helpful, have yet to supplant the wisdom of fleshly experience. What's bred in the bone will out, in time, for the prepared, attentive examiner.

But notice what my talk of reading and storytelling has done to Henry. In my role as physician, I've narrated his story, usurping his privilege of speaking in the first person. In writing his medical note, I make him an object of my knowing and recipient of my skill. I tell myself I've done this for the best of reasons and with his implicit consent: he came to me for help and I had to wrestle a story from his flesh. He wasn't going to share it in so many words. But what must I do to Henry to arrive at this place of useful knowing?

The word "diagnosis" comes from the Greek, *diagignoskein,* combining the verb meaning "to know" or "to learn," with the prefix *dia-*, variously translated as "through," "thoroughly," or "apart." It's a bit much for me to claim I "know thoroughly" someone I've only just met, while "to know through" renders Henry strangely translucent, and "to know apart," tosses him aside like the husk from an ear of roasted corn. None of the possible translations recognizes him as a person. The temptation accompanying the medical gaze is to confuse the physician's limited knowing with real insight into the person before me. To be clear, medical knowing needn't be oppressive. It's most often beneficial and welcomed. I do well, however, to remember that "the appendicitis in Room 12" has a complex story that exceeds my diagnostic powers. While diagnosing the patient's disease, I mustn't stop seeing him as a mystery, an occasion of wonder.

Even when understood as a limited way of knowing, diagnosis can become a consuming pursuit, rich enough to fill a career. Radiologists and pathologists have done just that for decades. There are Navajo *hataałiis*—traditional healers—who diagnose through crystal gazing, hand trembling, or listening to the desert wind. They then refer the sufferer to those who perform the proper ceremonies for each spiritual ailment: a shooting chant for injuries from lightning, an enemy way for contact with the dead. My profession, formed by a desire for scientific control, sees diagnosis as a prelude to material therapy, folding both tasks into a single practice.

An anxious father carried his child into the Emergency Department one night, just down the hall from where I met Henry. Even from across the room, the boy looked sick. There wasn't much history: frequent vomiting and diarrhea, fever, drinking poorly. Over the past day, he'd grown increasingly tired, and now was hard to arouse. We laid him on a table while nurses busily circled, checking vital signs and removing his loose clothing. At such a time, habits are allies. I looked, listened, touched—reading my way toward an understanding: stuporous exhaustion, racing pulse, doughy skin, the slow seeping of color back into his fingertips after I firmly pressed my own finger there.

"He doesn't look good," a nurse said, nudging me toward a quick assessment.

"He's in shock. Let's get moving," I said.

Neither of us was flaunting our diagnostic skills. In children, shock spills quickly into cardiac arrest and death. Our team, formed by long practice, responded immediately: an intravenous line, fluids given as fast as possible, medicines to treat the shock state and its cause. This is why we drill: simulating rare, disastrous events so that no one's forced to learn emergency actions when a life is truly at stake. We are what we repeatedly do. Character is revealed in habit.

What was necessary at the time, though—what the nurse and I collaborated in doing—was to put in words, so that everyone could hear, precisely where we were: "This is the country called 'shock.' Children can die here. By naming it, we now know what to do." The words were key. Having identified our starting place, we traveled as best we could toward safer ground, rescuing a child in the process.

Pediatrics is rarely so dramatic. A bleary-eyed mother brings her two-month old to my office for a morning appointment. He's sleeping now, but last night was another nightmare of fitful crying and restless fidgeting. Recalling countless nights fathering my inconsolable sons, I intuit the transitory hell mom and child have entered: colic. Still, I ask questions and perform the exam. As I suspect, what I find is quite normal. The stories I share of my own nights comforting sons in their colicky misery afford some credibility to the assessment and advice I offer the baby's mother. She and I take more time than I'd devote to a child's cold. I ask who helps her, how often she can take a break from parenting, describe tricks for calming a crying baby. Mostly I assure her this, too, shall pass, though not as quickly as she wishes. I'll remind her she can call if she has questions or concerns. I won't make her child better, but I can listen.

The astonishing thing is that I don't have to go looking for stories. A boy, a girl, comes to me and dies. Henry limps into my examining room and suffers me to interrogate his flesh. People seek me out to tell me stories I have no earthly right to hear. Mothers and fathers trust I will use them well, that I'll make their children better, and they make themselves terribly vulnerable in the process. To be a patient (the Latin root means "to suffer") is to be vulnerable: a woman shivers under a flimsy gown on a cold examining table, an awkward teen nervously tells me secrets he's hidden from his parents. Patients expose their bodies and intimate details in a position of great vulnerability. Modern, bowdlerized versions of the Hippocratic Oath or the Code of Geneva have lately dropped proscriptions on abortion and euthanasia, but it's still thought unethical for doctors to violate a patient's trust. Sometimes that trust must first be earned.

Three year-old Sean didn't want to see me. Neither did his parents, who'd spent the night dealing with Sean's fevered misery. Already exhausted, they were also angry our office hadn't called in an antibiotic for what they presumed was an ear infection. We avoid indiscriminately throwing antibiotics at our patients, but we're not particularly good at explaining why.

I wasn't in a good mood, either. Sean's appointment time was overbooked, an extra patient added to an already busy morning. By the time I entered the room I was well behind schedule. There would be no time to catch up over lunch, either. I had to use that time to round on inpatients. My quick apologies to Sean's parents for their wait went nowhere. In their eyes, I had made them wait for an unnecessary appointment. After a chilly conversation about Sean's illness, I'd moved on to the exam, but Sean's parents stayed in their chairs, staring at me with arms crossed, offering no help. I awkwardly pressed Sean's head to the examining table and peered into his ear with an otoscope, while the boy wriggled, kicked, and screamed. I quietly fumed at the couple's ingratitude. I was trying to help their son, and they were doing nothing to help me. Worse still, their diagnosis was correct. Sean had an ear infection after all, his right eardrum bulging in a dome of flaming red. When I released my head hold, Sean's foot swung up and caught me in the jaw.

I handed their furious son back to his parents, caught my breath, and described the ear infection I'd found. Sean's father, nodding quickly, said, "We already knew that."

I sat down to write the antibiotic prescription, my eyes focused on the pad of paper in front of me. I didn't want to look at them. I'd seen enough of their resentment to last me all day. And as I wrote, I felt the brush of a hand against my arm and heard the voice of Sean's mother, nearly silent until now. "Thank you," she said.

I looked up, toward the three of them. Sean's mother brought her left hand back to cradle the head of her child, sobbing softly in her lap. Sean's father was still visibly upset, but I heard for the first time his long, soft sighs of exhaustion. I asked how other things were going at home.

"Not so good," Sean's mother said. Nodding toward her husband, she continued, "David lost his job."

"Oh," I said. "I'm sorry."

We talked awhile longer, united at last in our shared concern for a sick boy, but I mostly listened, humiliated to rediscover how much I had to learn.

Doctors like to call the triumph of compassion over rage "professionalism." My mother called it loving kindness. Hard work, either way.

With Sean's family, it took a touch and a voice to help me remember where I was, what I was doing, whom I was with. Remember. Re-member. In these epiphanies, I exit the mind's airy palace and reclaim my body, assuming its neglected members: pulling on arms like gloves, my face snug as a woolen hat. I'm sure the body is smaller than the mind, the former built, by definition, to human scale. Suddenly the bodies I read and the stories I hear are no longer a series of puzzles to be solved or inconveniences to overcome, but embraceable mysteries. If it just happened more often.

"Only connect,"[1] E. M. Forster counsels, but I don't recall him saying how. Novelists like Forster are in the business of showing, not telling. Well into my struggle to make sense of seemingly irreconcilable callings: medicine, writing, family, and a spotty concern for the poor, I met up with a writer I'd come to know first through her books and then an exchange of emails. She was older than I, the mother of several nearly grown children, a former Professor of English Literature who ditched academics for motherhood. After what she called "a long and well-earned depression," she began a second career as an author of wise and learned books. It wasn't ready to leave medicine, but I longed to write, and I looked to her for guidance. I was anxious to speak with her at the conference in Chicago where our paths finally crossed, and she, sensing the busy convention hall was far from adequate for conversation, asked, "You want to go out for a beer?"

Over mugs of heady ale, we shared our struggles to fit writing into the messiness of our lives: academics and motherhood for her, medicine and fatherhood for me. Suddenly her brow furrowed, her eyes focusing on mine with new intensity. "So, do you regret becoming a doctor?" she asked.

I paused in a long, airy breath, thinking about bodies and words, how both staked their claims upon me, and how I longed to connect them. I could have abandoned medicine for writing, or storytelling for medicine, and my life would have been simpler, more coherent, and quite possibly happier. But neither choice was mine to make. What I sense in the body and what I discover on the page are tethered invisibly in me, joined by an umbilical cord, fashioned God knows how, when, or why. I ran my finger along the foam clinging to my glass and answered, at last, "I can't think of any other way I could have gotten to where I am now."

"Good," she said. "That's what I wanted to hear."

1. Forster, *Howard's End*, 174.

Chapter Six

Paying Attention

Departamento de Yoro,
Honduras/Grand Canyon, Arizona

WE SAT IN THE back of the pickup, saying little, staring at a mountain ridge
that rose through morning mist as if shedding a nightgown. Amy, who had
been in the country longer than the rest of us, said: "Honduras is so gorgeous at a distance. It's only when you get close that you see all the problems." Her words became a formula for understanding our experience. I had
been introduced the day before, on arrival in San Pedro Sula, to the trick of
spotting the telling detail. The airport there is well kept, surprisingly small
for the region's growing business center. I cleared passport control quickly,
and chatted with Miguel, one of our hosts, while we waited for the rest of
our group. After the usual questions about flights and weather, he pointed
to the airport's walls, made of crushed white rock. There, at a level just above
my chin, ran a continuous faint brown line, as if someone had pulled down
the wainscot but never touched up the paint. "That's how high the water was
after Mitch," he said solemnly, and I stepped to the wall for a closer look.

Everyone in Honduras knows "Mitch," the 1998 hurricane that came
from the Gulf and stalled overhead for an entire day, dropping nearly three
feet of rain on scarred, unstable land. What Mitch did to Honduras defies
comprehension: whole valleys flooded; roads washed away or buried by
landslides; farms, houses, families, lives—all gone. Mitch's rampage brought
me to Honduras, six months later. I came to help those in need. I also wanted

64

a change to keep my regular practice from growing stale. As much as I enjoyed children and looked forward to the next diagnostic mystery, a waiting room full of crying, stuffy-nosed, and diarrheal kids will lose its charm. I surrendered to the routine but came home exhausted, unable to give myself to my own children or my wife, much less my writing. This short-term medical service trip was an experiment, a scouting expedition into other forms of doctoring. I was a member of a twenty-four person medical team, the first since the hurricane to visit the village of San Jose, our destination in the highlands. It had taken five months just to reopen the dirt road, the only route from the mountains to the cities on the plain. We were among the first to test that road.

If there's a seat belt law in Honduras, it's not enforced. Crouching among suitcases in the back of the uncovered pickup, we had a pleasant, level ride across the valley toward the mountains. We raced past empty fields that had once been lush with banana trees, but I'd never seen the place before, and didn't know what to mourn. The wind played with my hair, and I laughed, glad the adventure had begun.

Things grew quiet as we left the highway to start the rough ascent. Houses—shacks, really—decayed under thick tree cover. Children waved as we passed. Barefoot boys battered a soccer ball through stick goalposts by the roadside. Parts of the route showed signs of recent construction, the ground disturbed, trees toppled. At places where the tropical forest thinned, we saw how abruptly the hillside fell away. Vultures circled in the updrafts. The Sula Valley disappeared. I leaned over the sideboard and looked down two hundred feet, sat down again and wedged myself more securely among the luggage. If we tipped, it was all over anyway, but I didn't want to be the fool launched overboard.

Higher up, farmers tend coffee—not in flat fields, but on those same crazy mountain slopes, storm-scoured and treacherous. North Americans wouldn't put up with this. I imagine they'd level the place, start over with wedding cake terraces reinforced with concrete and steel. Anything but this tragic resignation to topography. I don't think for a minute there's an inherent "closeness to the land" keeping Hondurans from remaking the world to their liking. The locals reshape things as much as the available technology permits. But technologies of power are expensive and available to few, none of whom live in these mountains.

The houses along the road grew in number, more solid, and we were suddenly there. A hand-painted banner over the town square announced: "*Bienvenidos*," and we felt welcome. The first half of our medical team had arrived well before, establishing our clinic in the schoolhouse. Time was short. We unloaded the truck, ate lunch at the Catholic Church, and began seeing patients. Patient they were: standing in line outside the schoolhouse gate, sitting in the hot sun between triage and clinic, enduring my limited Spanish and the wait for an available translator. At times someone from the pharmacy would walk into the room and announce: "We're already out of medicines for asthma," or "Ibuprofen is the only thing left for pain."

We had entered strange, disorienting territory, and I groped for something familiar with which to steady myself. Who better to consult than the "Founder of Modern Medicine" and champion of compassionate detachment, William Osler. A century ago, Dr. Osler—quoting the stethoscope-inventing Rene Laennec—told Johns Hopkins students: "Listen to the patient; he is giving you the diagnosis." Osler brought students to the patient's bedside and taught by example, master to apprentice, demonstrating techniques of medical historiography, careful listening, the art of the pertinent question. Then he would proceed to the examination, methodically searching for clues that give away the game. For future generations, he became the model attending: the senior physician whose signature habits are presence and attention. Modern medical education is so fundamentally Oslerian we can't fathom how revolutionary he was. In North America, Osler's success engendered its own subversion, the crisp certainty of machine data replacing sensuous impressions gathered by eyes, ears, and fingers. New and expensive tools don't merely enhance the older approach; they overwhelm it. Yet Osler remains the ghost in the clinical machine. His priests still murmur in shadowy side chapels of teaching hospitals. When fiscally-driven brevity and technological dazzle fail to cure, we invoke his spirit, return to half-forgotten ways. We learn again how one attends to the body at hand.

Lost in Honduras, I needed Osler's ghost. I suppose it came, real or imagined—a reassuring presence reminding me of rituals imperfectly abandoned. By mid-afternoon, my interpreter and I found a comfortable rhythm. She knew which questions came next. When I asked the unexpected, she threw me a surprised glance. She watched carefully as I examined patients. I'm no Osler, but I did my best. Crouching beside a trembling five-year-old, I peered at his eardrum, watched it flutter in a puff of air. Through my stethoscope, I listened for the soft murmur betraying his heart's secrets. My hand searched the hollow beneath his ribs for a swollen tip of spleen. In the end, spoon-shaped fingernails and the paleness around his eyes surrendered the diagnosis: severe iron deficiency anemia, probably worsened by parasitic infection. I wrote for iron pills and a liquid to cure him of worms, and told his mother the importance of bringing him back to the *Centro de Salud* when his iron ran out. I hoped there might be some pills left to give him if he came back.

Patients filed in one at a time, many silently announcing diagnoses from across the room: the vigilant, bewildered eyes of a man with schizophrenia; a long neglected fracture distorting a woman's forearm. Others brought subtler clues. A mother burdened by joint and muscle pains, given the chance to tell her story, was clearly depressed. The soft crackles heard in a girl's lungs explained her fevers: pneumonia. Some visitors left us mystified, their source of suffering yielding neither to our questions nor our touch. For them, we had little to offer: no subspecialists, no reassuring second opinions. What we had we gave: toothbrushes and bars of soap vitamins, and pills against the ubiquitous parasites.

Medical students approached me with other patients' stories, sharing in the ritual of history, physical, assessment, and plan. Always the familiar practice: we listen to a story, search for clues, propose a solution to the mystery, assist in the denouement. We had no laboratory, no electricity, few numbers to discuss. The crutches of industrial medicine were gone, leaving us little more than unaided senses. Grown men and women lay on schoolroom tables to be examined. Sheets hung from the ceiling, with little privacy for more intimate inspections. One doctor did minor surgery in a separate building, approximating as best he could aseptic technique and optimal anesthesia. People came, some walking three hours just to be seen, exposing to us their bodies and lives, sharing stories of illness, pain, untended wounds, malnourished children. No one mentioned Mitch unless asked—the eight hundred pound gorilla in the dirt-floored living room of their lives, best left undisturbed.

We found ways to talk of Mitch, usually outside the clinic walls. On an afternoon walk, I met an elderly woman who lost half her kitchen and all her vegetable crop to Mitch. She spoke softly, gently moving her fingertips over the smoke-stained fabric of her patchwork apron. A loose braid of gray hair fell over her right shoulder, her face so painfully expressive I could almost ignore the goiter—a sign of chronic iodine deficiency—bulging in her throat. "I have only poverty to look forward to," she said, then fell silent. Up the hill, her neighbor dried mud bricks in the sun, slowly rebuilding his house when away from his paying job: working another man's fields. The sturdiest home I visited belonged to a woman in her fifties whose husband had abandoned her ten years ago, leaving seven children to raise. Her boys, who now work in San Pedro, repaired her walls after the hurricane. She stood proudly with her daughters by a bed incandescent with *impatiens*, and worried aloud how soon the rich countries will forget about Mitch and Honduras will again ignore her village. On the wall by her front door, someone has written in chalk: "*Dios es amor! Cristo vive! Amen.*"

On our walk back to the clinic at the end of the day I asked Julio, a Honduran medical student and interpreter, what his government thought of these mountain people and their troubles. He looked at me a moment, his mouth frozen in a crooked half-smirk, before saying: "They don't." His answer was—to an extent—unjust. Honduran medical graduates must do a year of public health service, and there are some in power who work tirelessly for the poor. Yet Honduras is a land of entrenched disparity, as are many neighboring countries, including the United States. The Honduran elite are not alone in ignoring, whenever possible, the powerless.

I pressed Julio further: "How much has Mitch changed things?"

He smirked again. "Oh, Mitch. Mitch changed everything. But not as much as you might think."

I slowed, looked around me. Towering palms rose from a dense green thicket full of shrubs, birds, and insects I'd never seen before. Two men carrying machetes, their shirts sweat-soaked from a long day in the sun, preceded us on the dusty path winding upward to the village. A road full of ruts and furrows slashed through low brush toward a single house on the next ridge. Beyond, the mountains basked in evening light. I was glad to be here, glad in a terribly selfish way that Mitch had brought me to this place, though I knew Mitch was only another sad chapter in a much longer story.

I turned back to Julio, still watching me with apparent amusement. "Sorry," I muttered, picking up the pace.

We would be late for dinner.

In the evenings after clinic closed, children visited us in the schoolyard. The girls seemed astonished by our attention. They tossed fluorescent yo-yos while the boys beat the medical students in soccer. I grew particularly fond of Cristia: tall, silent, with short, black curls and a luminous smile. She had an unaffected modesty absent in countries where children wallow in television and spectacle. A look of sorrow lingered a moment after someone caught her eye, then died in a blossoming grin. I spoke to her in lame Spanish, discovering only that she was eleven years old, born on the feast of *La Virgen de Guadalupe*, and had never traveled far from her village. On the day we left, I told her I would miss seeing her. She smiled, said nothing, and looked shyly away.

I guessed the details of her life. She was tall, meaning her family was able to feed her. They had a little money; she wore a well-mended pink dress. Like most of her friends, she spent the day barefoot and was probably infected with hookworm, among other parasites, burrowing through unprotected skin to steal her blood. I never met her family, never found her home. She disappeared with the other children at dusk as the schoolyard gate closed, locking us in, the villagers out. Night settled slowly, the forest swelled with the unearthly screech of insects, and the street emptied, save the usual parade of dogs, pigs, and chickens.

The parade was still there at sunrise. Sows with dripping dugs nosed debris along the fence. Roosters, who'd been crowing since shortly after midnight, chased hens in the underbrush. The children returned, too, busy with chores. A boy hacked a log with a machete. Another carried a heavy rifle on his shoulder. Girls passed with purposeful elegance, holding bowls of corn meal or pails of water.

Each morning that week, I looked across the misty valley to the mountains of Yoro, and whispered the words of the bride in San Juan de la Cruz's "Spiritual Canticle": "*Mi Amado, las montanas . . . .*"[1] Each morning I watched the mountains undress for the day, felt again the tearing apart of this beautiful world, remembered how much suffering lived here, was quietly borne here, in this cruel Eden. We had come to change that, bring it under our control, armed with book learning, donated medicines, and the best of intentions. But what were we doing, patching up bodies in a mountain village, when an entire country lay in ruins? A few doctors gathered by candlelight after sundown and shared grand plans, bold solutions for Honduras's problems. They were full of energy, more likely than I to make something important happen.

Yet, as the days in the clinic sped by, I realized our Honduran patients were offering me a gift. This confused me. They were in no position to be generous. They had no obligation to welcome me into their pain. They knew how little I could do to make things better. They seemed less interested in curative therapy than in having someone hear their story, attend to their pain, bear witness to their suffering. Their tacit recognition of my impotence shamed me, though never openly nor deliberately. Truth hid in the uncertain silence between words, the calluses of a hand offered in friendship, the sorrow masked in a smile. No doubt I missed a great deal, but I was grateful for the gifts I recognized. I held them till they hatched unexpected questions. Here's one: If the particulars of their pain were merely problems awaiting solution, why did touching that pain, if only for a moment and largely on my own terms, make me feel lighter, more at home in the world, so far away from all I called home?

* * * *

---

1. St. John of the Cross, *Canciones entre el alma y el esposo*, in *The Poems of St. John of the Cross*, 102.

I have another home. Not where I live now, but one before all that: the desert, my heart's true landscape. That's where I started to learn how medical practice informed my entire life: how the rituals of listening, examination, and diagnosis schooled me in practices of attention—not just toward bodies, but the whole world.

Walking home from the hospital after a day of few victories and all too many lessons in humility, I would stop to look at the land. The Moenkopi plateau sloped upward to the southeast, shimmering in the heat, ripples of red and gray under a sky so blue it hurt to watch. To the south rose the San Francisco Peaks, snow-laced extinct volcanoes the Navajo name *Dook'o'ooslííd,* Sacred Mountain of the West, and the Hopi say are home to the *katsinam,* beneficent spirits who bring the desert people rain. "I live here," my heart would sing, "This is my home, too."

Vastness, capricious erosion, blessed silence: these are some of the desert's gifts. There are desert places I visit just to be quiet and alone. The readiness is all. I once rested atop Hunt's Mesa after a hard climb and looked on Monument Valley below: alien as an arctic waste, sandstone icebergs drifting in waterless red seas. A single raven flew out beyond the rim, rising suddenly on a current of air. I heard each beat of her wings as she passed. Another time I'd have missed that gift, lost in sterile self-absorption. Simone Weil, in her essay on the right use of school studies, asserts: "Never . . . is a genuine effort of the attention wasted."[2] Students of fierce landscapes will, I think, agree.

The desert is a barren, inhospitable place to those who haven't yet learned to look closely, to find living treasures in this ocean of seeming lifelessness. Once Jill and I walked the south rim of Grand Canyon, having hiked the day before from our camp at river level. We moved with the achy shuffle of canyon greenhorns. A cold front moved in, and we watched icy cloud fingers test the rocky edge before probing the abyss. A well-dressed couple walking in the other direction stopped us a moment and asked, "Does the view get any better up ahead?" We told them "no," which was the truth. It didn't get better anywhere unless you went in, got closer, saw things on the scale in which they're lived.

Who has time for that? I live in the city now, where it's work to slow down and see. Were I caught up in the tourists' rush to the gift shop, would I want to learn about outrageous life thriving just over the rim? Would I pause to hear the agave's story: how it sends towering flower spikes to heaven after years of slow growth, pollinating, seeding and dying in one brief season of

2. Weil, "Reflections on the Right Use of School Studies with a View to the Love of God," in *Waiting for God,* 106.

glory, leaving behind ghostly staffs, sentinels in the desert wind? Would I stay to watch the gray-feathered water ouzel wading canyon creeks improbably named Bright Angel, Clear, or Crystal, dipping in and out of chill water as if doing calisthenics? Would I want to see the tiny insects he scoops in his bill, devouring other life to keep his own? Would I stop planning my next vacation long enough to notice the tiny white bundles clinging to the prickly pear which, when rubbed with a stick, burst in a brilliant flourish of reddish-purple?

Spanish newcomers wandered these deserts centuries ago, looking for—among other things—these bundles of cochineal to color fine fabrics. The Spanish who stayed grew used to desert rhythms. They saw more carefully than I do. They looked on life and death without flinching, not taking refuge in myths of ease and control. Their descendants, like Osler's priests, inhabit twilight margins. They labor in the shadow of the Sangre de Cristo mountains, attend to the desert's harsh tutelage, know the terrible price of hurry and inattention. They see their grandchildren and those of their Anglo neighbors devoured by beautiful American illusions: the narcotic of entertainment, the lure of a fast life, the illusion of a painless one.

I, in turn, learned to love Grand Canyon's instructive immensity, visiting as often as possible. The Canyon remains a necessary part of any return to the Reservation, a contemplative touchstone, a pilgrimage. I once spent a week hiking rim-to-rim with Wayne, a geologist friend of mine who'd been a backcountry ranger for the National Park Service. On a brilliant October morning, we shouldered our packs as ravens cackled advice from the pines. Our starting place was the South Rim and shortest route to the other side was down. "We're going to go slow," he said, "Take our time. See what you might otherwise walk past." I'd hiked the canyon before and led trips myself. I was content to let him set the pace.

The lessons began almost immediately. Shortly after beginning our descent, he pointed out Indian pictographs I'd unknowingly walked past many times. Further in, he showed me an Ancestral Puebloan ruin hidden from the trail, its centuries-old walls decaying in the shadow of a cliff overhang. In the nearby sand lay the skeleton of a mule deer, picked clean yet almost perfectly articulated, as if the flesh had simply dissolved where the body had fallen. It was so quiet, I half expected our conversation and the crunch of gravel underfoot to rouse ghosts from long fallow gardens of squash and corn. We moved on, exploring unconformities: places in the rock where strata of very different ages abut and huge chunks of history have been lost. We talked about geologic time, human time, the spiral of seasons, and we walked, always downward, always closer to the river at the center of the world.

Shedding the packs at our first campsite, we scrambled to a nearby cliff edge and looked down on the swirling Colorado, not a muddy red as its name suggests but eerily green. Upstream, Glen Canyon Dam traps millions of tons of iron-rich sediment daily, while clear, cold reservoir-bottom water flows into the canyon below. Only after heavy rain does the river blush again, muddied by runoff. We were drawn to the river, but we knew we'd sleep tonight on this flat shelf known as the Tonto Platform, the halfway point in our vertical descent.

The Tonto is one of the world's classic sequences of sedimentary rock, divided by geologists into three layers: Muav Limestone, Bright Angel Shale, and Tapeats Sandstone. They chronicle the eastward movement of an ocean shoreline over the course of twenty million years during the Cambrian period, ending some 500 million years ago. Paleontologists describe the Cambrian as a dreamtime of wonderful, often bizarre life blossoming in marine shallows, the biological origins of all that followed and much that vanished along the way. In the waning afternoon light, on a gentle slope where the sandstone blurs into greenish shale, Wayne and I looked for trace fossils: trails, burrows, and other remnants of ancient animal life, the invertebrate equivalent of dinosaur tracks. Paired holes in the rock are thought to have been made by burrowing creatures in the soft offshore bottoms. Ruffles in the stony surface are said to be trilobite tracks. It took considerable imagination to envision a thriving undersea community in the vanished Tapeats Sea. The pleasant images I conjured: undulating reefs of coral, white breakers on immaculate beaches, were undoubtedly more Caribbean than Cambrian.

We returned to camp as the light failed. Even in October, the inner canyon was sufficiently warm and mosquito free for us to forgo tents and spread the sleeping bags on the sand. It's a treat not to be missed, lying under desert stars as they circle Polaris in a cosmic pavane. I once read that Francis of Assisi saw the universe as literally dependent, hanging from the Creator like so many tendrils from a great tree. It's an odd image for moderns, so certain which way is up that a former Vice President of the United States is rumored to have complained to *The Washington Post* that an image of earth from space printed in their pages was "upside down."[3] The story may be apocryphal, if plausible to generations used to finding the North Pole at the top of any map of the world. The real question, however, is, "Upside down relative to what?" Francis was on to something: we hang from above, invisibly connected to everything that is. As I lay in my sleeping bag looking into the rest of the universe, details of the Milky Way shone in crisp focus. No

3. It is alleged that Al Gore, Jr. made a call to the *Washington Post*'s executive editor, Leonard Downie, Jr., in March, 1998, to express his concern about the photo.

wonder the ancients believed stars shaped human destiny. Contemplating such immensity should humiliate the most confirmed narcissist and undermine illusions of autonomy. It might even compel me to accept a place, however small, in the lower reaches of a pendulous universe.

The canyon is like a mountain upside-down, as if some titan had pressed a long, sinuous ridge into the Colorado Plateau, leaving behind the trough we now descend to reach where once lay the summit. Our vertical drop from South Rim to River approximates a mile, broken up by cliffs and slopes along which the narrow footpath writhes. Slopes are rather easy to traverse, while cliffs require wriggling switchbacks, some with names like "Devil's Corkscrew" or "Jacob's Ladder." Perhaps the biggest barrier to foot traffic in the Grand Canyon is the Redwall Limestone, a consistent cliff 400 to 600 feet high running just above the Tonto Platform. We had negotiated the Redwall's switchbacks our first day, and as dawn pointed beyond the rim on Day Two, I spied Venus—the Morning Star—in a niche of the Redwall to the east. The cool morning tempted us to linger, but we ate quickly and began hiking, anxious to reach the river before the sun heated the inner canyon. More switchbacks awaited. We were glad to be going down. I heard a canyon wren sing a cheery falling scale ending in a squawk. We breached the rim of the Tonto, occasionally glimpsing the Colorado as we descended the inner gorge. Then, unexpectedly, we were at the river itself. For me there is no better place, with all the world above, the sound of the river within, and all around, my favorite rock in the world: Vishnu Schist.

One of my Grand Canyon books describes the metamorphic rock of the Vishnu as "mostly foliated mica schist," a bit like calling the Sistine Chapel a painted church. It's not that the Vishnu Schist is classically beautiful, like polished marble, or brilliant, like a freshly opened geode. The Vishnu varies in color from gray to black, studded with tiny crystals formed millions of years ago in the heart of a long vanished mountain range. It's this stars-in-the-sky appearance that compels me to touch the rock and run my hands along its rippled surface. Bizarre fractures and knobby eroded forms mimic living organisms. Whenever I hear the cliché, "carved from the living rock," I picture the Vishnu. Yielding grudgingly to water's destructive force, this very thick, very hard stone forms steep, craggy slopes that fracture along fine striations—the "planes of foliation"—rising vertically from the shore. White quartz ripples like taffy through the midnight sky of stone, while in other places, tiny garnets glisten in the sun. Fingers of pink Zoroaster Granite splay out through the schist, remnants of magma pockets that cooled a billion and a half years ago. If that seems too much time to grasp, consider that the Vishnu Schist is five hundred million years older, nearly the oldest exposed rock on the planet.

I have a passing acquaintance with basic principles of geology, including ways in which rocks are dated. Yet I suspect no amount of study, no degree of understanding, prepares the brain to comprehend two billion years. What part of my experience touches such enormity? Except for corporate budgets or destruction done by hurricanes, why talk about billions of anything? The number's too big, and we never get close enough to understand. Yet I can touch the Vishnu Schist, and know I'm in the presence of mystery.

Albert Einstein once observed: "The most beautiful emotion we can experience is the mystical. It is the source of all true art and science. He to whom this emotion is a stranger, who can no longer wonder and stand rapt in awe, is as good as dead."[4] I hate to quibble with Einstein, but the mystical is more than an emotion. Mystical experience certainly has an emotional component, though it is also a way of perception, a close, attentive encounter with that which resists explanation. Einstein is surely right, however, in saying the sciences are no enemy of mystery. Science often sharpens mystery, even as it explains, revealing startling symmetries and rendering the commonplace rich and strange. I touch the Vishnu Schist much as I read Shakespeare, in awe and wonder. Great science, like great works of art, "pass(es) through us like storm winds, flinging open the doors of perception, pressing down upon the architecture of our beliefs with their transforming power."[5] So writes George Steiner (about works of art, not science), and despite the broadened meaning I give his words, I'm with him a hundred percent. But I should finish my story.

The next day, after tidying up the breakfast things and filling our water bottles, we began a day hike up to a great view and the Great Unconformity, the geological dividing line between the 500 million year old rocks of the Tonto Platform and much older layers below. Our path was a narrow trail used more often by foraging mule deer than by humans—it rose in steep switchbacks up the Vishnu, then across talus slopes of intermediately aged rock layers named Bass Limestone, Hakatai Shale, and Shinumo Quartzite. As we ascended, I recited their names softly, rolling them on my tongue like rich Bordeaux. In first year of medical school, I memorized the twelve cranial nerves using common mnemonics: sentences—some silly, others salacious—in which each successive word began with the same letter as the corresponding nerve. Here, though, in the presence of these strata, I needed no memory aid. To know their names was an intellectual pleasure. To apprehend their beauty directly with my eyes, hands, and feet, was joyful participation.

4. Einstein, as quoted by Patrick, *Introduction to Philosophy*, 44.
5. Steiner, *Tolstoy Or Dostoevsky*, 3.

The trail over the steepening rock slope faded away, though I could see where we were headed: toward a break in the Tapeats Sandstone through which we could reach the plateau. The closer we came, the more we scrambled over boulders, at first the size of cars, then living rooms, then houses. We stopped often to rest and sip our water. Near the cleft, we climbed in shadow. Our breaks grew longer and more silent, perhaps from the somber light, perhaps because we were simply out of breath. Once over the rim, we returned to full sunlight. Wayne refilled his canteen from a pothole brimming with last week's rain. We stood exhausted, silently taking in the sweep of the river below, its barely audible rapids still enlarging the canyon.

Suddenly Wayne grew visibly excited. He pointed to a part of the canyon where the rock bed is jumbled, near the Great Unconformity where Precambrian Shinumo Quartzite boulders appear in the much younger Tapeats Sandstone. Rocks of such different ages don't usually mix that way. Wayne explained how the quartzite had formed islands in the Tapeats sea half a billion years ago, the same waters in which trilobites scuttled to make the tracks we'd seen two days before. Some of those quartzite islands eroded away in the surf. Boulders tumbled from island cliffs into the sea, settling in a sandy bottom that slowly petrified around them. Millions of years later, they were exposed by the carving of the canyon. As Wayne described it, the image assembled in my mind. That ancient fall into surging tide was, unlike so much of the canyon's history, a moment I could picture in human scale, within experience, a recognizable detail captured in the vastness of geologic time. I asked him if finding such a tiny thing, so amazing, so connected with the breaking apart and rising up of our own life, was like making some great discovery, like unearthing the ruins of Troy. "No," he said, turning to face me directly, squinting in the bright sun: "It's like seeing God."

Chapter Seven

Affections

Tuba City, Navajo Nation

THE WINDOW BLINDS FINALLY pushed Jill over the edge. What she wanted seemed reasonable enough: a set of window blinds for the conference room at the far end of the pediatric unit. As it was, when someone projected a video or slides there during a meeting, pinned-up bed sheets masked just enough direct desert sunlight to approximate high noon on an overcast day. Cotton sheets served passably for the medical staff, used as we were at making do with scarcity. The dynamics changed when Jill planned a conference of obstetricians and midwives from around the state. She wanted the conference room dark enough for slide presentations to be more than ghostly images projected on a white wall, and with means more professional in appearance than bed sheets and safety pins. It didn't seem a luxury, but in an era of federal budget slashing, that's what it was called.

Buying and installing window blinds requires planning and precision in any case, but the maze through which Jill had to navigate to avoid even the appearance of wasting taxpayer dollars was long, cumbersome, and slow. In practice—and perhaps by design—the process punished action. Approval and procurement takes weeks. Jill didn't have weeks, so she drove to the Sears store in Flagstaff with measurements in hand, and bought them. With her own money. That alone constituted procedural overreach. Federal regulations further required any installer be federally approved, again to avoid hint of waste. Scheduling an approved installer to drive to a small desert town takes weeks and a tidy sum of cash, the latter requiring official approval before funds are designated and released. Jill made another end run around the regulations and talked one of the Hopi maintenance men into doing the job. He took several days, but finished in time for the conference. In the end, the room looked reasonably professional, Jill wasn't court-martialed, and the Feds saved money. To this day, when inspirational posters or motivational speakers share some pabulum about the journey trumping the destination, I think of Jill and the odyssey of the blinds. And then I sigh.

Though it was, in itself, a small incident, it marked a crescendo in my wife's occupational frustration. As seasoned clinicians finished their public service commitments and moved away to more lucrative or prestigious jobs, Jill had received the hospital equivalent of a battlefield promotion to chief of obstetrics and gynecology. She now dealt regularly with federal budget constraints, a frustrating bureaucracy, talented but fractious colleagues, and an endless loop of physician recruitment and replacement. The slow loss of good people was nothing new. When we first arrived in Tuba City to work, we signed on for two years, at the end of which we re-upped for two more. We would add a fifth year before leaving, but the possibility of leaving grew less theoretical, an expectation rather than one option among many.

While Jill had her bureaucratic dark night of the soul, I mired myself in another round of professional self-interrogation. The problem wasn't medicine itself, which was a good in my life, but not the only good. Life's turf battles rarely pit good against bad. More often, they're about relative goods. St. Augustine named the challenge of deciding between relative goods the *Ordo Amoris*: the order of loves. For Augustine, human suffering isn't the natural consequence of desire itself, but what comes of attending to our loves in the wrong order, honoring lesser affections before greater ones, or misdirecting desires in destructive ways, like an addict hoping his next fix will satisfy—once and for all—the gnawing emptiness in his chest. As for me, medicine, writing, marriage, and fatherhood bobbed in a sea of relative goods. My challenge was to keep from clinging to any one too dearly, lest the swirling flotsam drag me under. Medicine was a good in my life, and it paid quite a few bills. I had no intention of quitting my day job, but writing was a good, too.

If writing had been nearly as important to me as I said, I would have found the self-discipline to make it happen. Instead, I played at the craft, talked about what I'd do if I found enough uninterrupted hours, and showed more interest in having written than in sitting in a chair long enough to put one sentence after another on the page before me. I had no recognizable work ethic. Rather than building one, I blamed myself: right target, wrong response.

One evening, after I came home from the hospital to hole up in a room with a book, Jill said, "You know, our kids need you, too, Brian. I need you. You come home exhausted, and we don't see a smile, never hear a story about what went right today, or share the cheerfulness you show your patients. You mutter something from the door before you head upstairs with a book, and by the time I can talk to you, you're asleep. We need your attention. How can we get you back?"

I reluctantly admitted she was right. The two of us devised a plan to cut my time at the hospital by one day a week, affording me a regular "writing day" and freeing the hospital to hire another pediatrician to meet growing patient numbers and needs. It was a worthy experiment. I used the time to write, if never as efficiently or consistently as I might have. Still, I was cheered at making some progress. Jill, too, seemed happier between her jousts with bureaucracy. My encounters with patients and the stories they shared remained, for the most part, tangible joys.

* * * *

EDNA CARED FOR OUR sons while Jill and I worked at the hospital. She had watched over the children of several doctors before us and raised nine of her own in one-room house in the Hopi village across the highway. The Hopi live in villages on mesas above their fields, their lands surrounded by the much larger Navajo reservation. Hopis, like Navajos, transfer property along maternal lines, so the house where Edna lived—and often took our boys—belonged to her and not her husband, Walter. Walter farmed a plot in the valley below the village. Though he'd worked the same ground since returning from the Korean War, he always called it "Effie's field." Effie was Walter's mother-in-law. By Hopi tradition the farmland belonged to Effie and would pass to Edna or Edna's daughters upon her death.

Edna's daughters devoted themselves to educational opportunities denied their parents, earning graduate degrees before returning home to teach at local schools. Her sons were less ambitious, holding intermittent jobs supplemented with cash earned selling *katsina* figures—painted sculptures of Hopi spirit beings—they carved from cottonwood root. When the boys ran afoul of the law, crashed a truck on the highway, or got into a fight, Edna and Walter supported them and welcomed them back, almost without question. For Hopis, family trumps behavior. Always.

Edna loved to cook and loved watching others eat her food. Her mastery at the stove outstripped her command of English. She had a gift for skewed phrases, like "more better," or "you need some furnitures in here."

One of her daughters married a man with a Hispanic surname, and Edna cooked beans by the potsful whenever they came to visit, explaining, "Mexicans like beans, you know." Another time she told Jill, "Your kids like my cooking because I make everything with grease." I've every reason to believe that, at least, was true.

The boys joined our lives to Edna's: a shared love often expressed opaquely. Edna lectured Jill on proper baby care, pointing out our parental deficiencies wherever she found them. Her concerns included the universal childcare staples: sleep, temperature, and poop. When we fell short of her standards, she challenged us with prosecutorial fervor: "I can tell your baby slept cold last night. Look, his stool is green," displaying the evidence on a dirty diaper. I'd return home on a wintry evening after a day's work at the hospital to find the thermostat set to a steamy eighty degrees and our son asleep under extra blankets, layers of socks nested on his feet like Russian dolls. My years of pediatric training and Jill's mountain of parenting books meant nothing to Edna, who spoke from her own considerable experience. We came, in time, to accept that Will and Peter were as much her boys as ours. She loved them with a ferocity that more than compensated for her quaint opinions.

What's more, she welcomed us to her world, giving Will and Peter Hopi names and opening her home during village ceremonies. For Edna, hospitality was both discipline and joy. As our first *Powamu*, the Hopi Bean Dance held in early February, approached, she issued strict orders: be at her house before sunrise on the first day of the festival with our son warmly dressed for a morning outside. We did as instructed, Will thickly cocooned in his car seat as we drove to the lower village under a canopy of winter stars. At the time, the lower village where Edna lived was off the power grid, the sky unmarred by electric lines and utility poles. We descended the narrow dirt road from the more modern upper village and entered another time: kerosene lamps glimmered through tiny widow panes; small fires, banked overnight, sweetened the air with pinyon smoke; shadowy figures moved between adobe dwellings. If not for the occasional pickup truck parked along the way, we could imagine ourselves in the nineteenth century.

Edna's stone and adobe house shone at the farthest end of the downward road, its interior lighting powered by a grumbling kerosene generator. We parked, and entered with our son and a bag of fruit in tow—one learns not to arrive without a gift of food, no matter how small. The house, awash with family members and already quite warm, had a heater in one corner and pots of coffee and *Noquivi,* a traditional hominy and mutton stew, steaming on the gas stove. We let Edna serve us breakfast—one learns to accept hospitality when offered—and cleared the dishes as the eastern sky brightened.

The remainder of the day overflowed with gifts: traditional Hopi toys for our sons, presented to us on the main village plaza at sunrise; visitations from the benevolent and sometimes terrifying *katsinam*; *katsina* dances on the plaza; and, always, more food. Edna glowed with delight as her blending families shared stories around the table. Edna's work wasn't done when the festival ended. She would cook long hours afterward, returning favors extended her by others through "paybacks"—usually in the form of food—handed back and forth in slowly diminishing amounts over the next several weeks.

Edna's daughters showed little desire to make *piki*, the labor-intensive, paper-thin corn delicacy at the heart of Hopi hospitality rituals and "paybacks." Their disinterest broke a long chain, a loss unlikely to be redeemed. To watch a Hopi grandmother kneeling before a hot, flat stone in a cramped, smoky house, conjuring handfuls of watery corn mush into rolls of *piki,* is to stand in the presence of a master. The atmosphere is profoundly contemplative: wordless gestures and prayerful silence punctuated by the crinkle of coals glowing under a glistening *piki* stone. The resulting delicate rolls of crisp corn aren't particularly tasty to Anglo mouths trained to crave salt, but the world's a better place with *piki* makers in it.

To complain about *piki's* taste—its lack of salt or distinct note of wood ash—is to miss the point. *Piki* is a gift, passed between Hopi women in calibrated amounts, knitting persons into a community, nourishing new generations with old ways. Even that hint of ash lurking in the flavor is nourishing. Wood ash, intentionally added to the corn mush before baking, improves *piki's* nutritional value and reduces fungal toxins: a centuries-old indigenous practice called nixtamalization, in which corn is steeped with alkali, like ash or limewater. Not until the twentieth century did Anglos discover why a steady diet of unalkalinized corn leads to Pellagra, a disfiguring condition caused by a deficiency in the B vitamin, niacin, or from lack of certain amino acids. There's niacin in untreated corn, but not in a form available for human digestion. Nixtamalization frees the niacin and improves amino acid balance. Though Edna's ancestors didn't grasp the biochemistry, they knew what to do, and taught their children accordingly.

Where tradition and community are essential to survival, they are passed on through all possible means. The Hopi and Navajo languages, while unrelated, are both fabulously wealthy with terms of relationship. Family ties outweigh individual identities. Our son would return from a day at Edna's house with tales of what "*Vava*" had said or done, and though we recognized the Hopi word for "brother," precisely which of Edna's sons

Will meant was rarely clear. Native identity roots in the soil of genealogy and gender. In Hopi, there are very different words for "thank you," depending on whether the speaker is male or female. In Navajo, there's no generic "mother" or "grandmother," but there is "*shimá*" ("*my* mother") and "*shimá sani*," ("*my* grandmother"), in the same way there are words for *my* father and grandfather, *my* younger brother and older brother, *my* younger sister, and, yes, *my* older sister.

A Navajo introduces herself by naming the clan she is born to (her mother's clan) and for (her father's clan). All members of her mother's clan are considered first-degree relatives—brother or sister, mother or father—leading to English-language combinations, like "cousin-brother," sufficiently opaque to *bilagáanas* to bewilder a master of protocol. Traditional language resists modern forgetfulness, reminding speakers that identity is less *who* you are than *whose* you are. Relatedness and tradition filled the air Jill and I breathed, like the scent of burning pinyon at *Powamu*, a background of which we were, at best, intermittently aware.

* * * *

We lived as a statistical minority in a reservation town. Jill and I had grown up as unexceptionable white kids in homogeneous suburbs where everyone looked pretty much the same, the world consistently rewarded intelligence and hard work, and history happened long ago, somewhere else, and to other people. In Tuba City, we were conspicuously pale, couldn't help but see how ethnicity and class shaped success in life, and lived and worked with inheritors of brutal historical events that were anything but over.

Living as guests on Indian land, we were treated by our hosts far better than white people historically treated them. Still, no matter how long we stayed, we would never become native to the place. Institutions where non-Natives played a significant role—the hospital, churches, schools, and businesses—had seen too many outsiders arrive with transformative plans for the town and, after a brief, meteoric career of unsettling, unsustainable, and often unhelpful change, leave forever. Whatever the Navajo and Hopi people lacked, it wasn't newcomers with book learning, city smarts, and messianic schemes. I learned to listen long and well before offering solutions to other people's problems.

Even that didn't come easy. I grew accustomed to playing the inescapably rude Anglo. My Navajo friends appropriately pegged me as one more culturally disadvantaged *bilagáana*, and seemed amused, even surprised, whenever I apologized for my latest cultural faux pas. They figured I simply didn't know any better. There is, in fact, no idiomatically Navajo way to say "I'm sorry," no standard apology in the Navajo language. When I asked a Navajo healer how that could be, he said, "When a child is clumsy, the parent may say '*hozho*,' [Navajo for 'beauty,' 'harmony,' or 'balance,'] to remind him to get back in balance with the world. There's no way to say 'I'm sorry' in Navajo, because it's assumed you were raised properly and should know better. You should have learned in childhood."

If traditional Navajos rarely apologize, they love a good laugh. Words that sound very different in English may be distinguished from one another in Navajo by slight variations in tone, stress, or syllable length—fertile ground for puns. The same Navajo healer once stopped me in the middle of a conversation about *k'é*, the all but unfathomable Navajo word for "relationship." Grinning, he explained, "I know what you mean, but every time you try to say, '*k'é*,' you're actually saying the Navajo word for 'shoe.'"

My attempts at spoken Navajo frequently resulted in group laughter. When I asked what I'd gotten wrong in the language, I was told, "It's too funny to even tell you, Dr. Volck." Navajo humor tends toward knowing self-mockery, a reminder that everyone takes a turn at playing the fool. Good humor covers a multitude of sins, and it was a privilege to live, work, and raise a family with welcoming people when the unresolved sadnesses of their history should have made it otherwise. I had just enough self-awareness not to crow about my being a minority in a majority non-white town, if only because Jill and I—and everyone else—knew we were there by choice and could leave at anytime.

One evening at dinner, Will tried to explain the funny thing one of the kids at preschool had said, and I asked him who, precisely, the joker in question was. Without a pause, Will replied, "The one who's all brown," moving his open palm in front of his face for emphasis, as if he knew his own skin was too pale to convey his meaning. I asked him to be more specific, to give another clue, but all Will did was repeat the rubbing motion and say, "the one who's all brown." I pointed out to him that, with one or two exceptions, everyone in his preschool class was "all brown."

Another evening, Jill asked me if I'd noticed how Blondie, our reservation rescue mutt, growled and barked louder at Navajos than whites. I didn't believe Jill at first, but close observation proved her right, leaving me to puzzle what, if anything, in our behavior led our dog to fear humans who didn't resemble us. It was shameful, I thought, a behavior I tried, without success, to make him unlearn. The dog realized long before I that we weren't Indian.

If I wasn't Indian, who or what was I? Ready answers proved unsatisfying. Any response to the question, "Who am I?" was more complicated than I could articulate. From what the Navajo and Hopi had shown me, any legitimate answer includes heritage and ancestry. Perhaps I needed to return to my roots. Perhaps our children needed to hear their grandparents' stories straight from the source, spend more than a few random hours in the houses where Jill and I had grown up, and learn that they, too, came from a place, a time, and a people.

In the winter of our fifth year on the Rez, the year I was taking "a day off each week to write," several threads of awareness wove together: my discontent with medicine and longing to write, Jill's frustration with bureaucracy, and our lessons in the fragile necessity of tradition, lineage, and identity. Peter was still too young to express an opinion, but Will would start Kindergarten the following year. He was also discovering, if only on family vacations, that he had cousins, something he'd assumed unique to "all brown" kids. As Jill and I talked about where we might go after the Rez, our options quickly narrowed to two: Baltimore, where all Jill's family lived, or Cincinnati, with my parents and most of my siblings. Baltimore was, for Jill, the Promised Land she longed to reclaim. I had left Cincinnati at the end of high school with the sense that I was moving on, away, and for good.

Though Jill was readier than I to leave, I agreed it was time. We were surprised when our most appealing job offers came from Cincinnati. Jill found a university appointment, while I took a primary care position at an inner city health center on the Kentucky side of the Ohio River. As word spread that we were moving on, people at the hospital were quite kind, asking us why we were leaving after what seemed to them so short a time. When I answered, "Because our kids need to see their grandparents more than once or twice a year," our Navajo and Hopi friends would almost invariably lean closer, touch my shoulder with feathery lightness, and grin, sometimes adding, "Looks like we actually taught you something."

"Yes," I said, with an equally bittersweet grin, "Yes, you did."

On a clear July morning, we loaded up the car. The rising waves of sadness I stifled before they burst into sobs caught me by surprise. Jill and I had long since made our decision, enjoyed a succession of gracious farewell gatherings, and looked forward to the next chapter in our life and work. I imagined myself reconciled to leaving good friends, a landscape I'd come to love, and the place where my children were born. Now the children were in their car seats, flanking the dog that crouched in the middle, with a mountain of luggage and camping equipment behind them, and my chest felt hollow, evacuated of everything but sorrow. There was nothing to be done about it. We exchanged hugs, said our last goodbyes, and pulled away, past the houses of dear friends, past the hospital, past the drooping cottonwood trees along Main Street, and onto the highway heading east.

Chapter Eight

Vulnerabilities

Cincinnati, Ohio

OUR MOVE WASN'T ALL existential dread. We made a vacation out of the cross-country drive, camping and visiting friends along the way. When we arrived in Cincinnati, my family helped us move in and fed us as we set up house. Jill's parents visited soon thereafter, delighted at the shortened travel time required to see their grandchildren. We settled into new rhythms of neighborhood and work for us, school for Will, and childcare for Peter. The boys came to know their relatives better—aunts, uncles, and cousins—and made new friends. We visited my parents regularly, where Will and Peter heard family stories and my mother coached them in the telling of jokes. Having a joke for Grandma—new or retold didn't matter—became the token price of admission to her table. Will worked on delivery and timing. Peter improvised yarns about Mickey Mouse and Tyrannosaurus Rex meeting by chance in the woods, the humor of which was apparent to Peter, if not always to us. That the boys—and, later, our daughter—became accomplished joke tellers was a source of pride to my mother, who wrote jokes into her funeral plans as a last opportunity to share a lifelong joy.

Jill and I threw ourselves into new jobs. The clinic had continuities with the Indian Health Service hospital in Tuba City, poverty and limited resources among them—as well as surprising differences. The inner city is grittier than the desert: more corrosive to its poorest inhabitants and, despite its population density, far more isolating. From appearances, the unrelieved harshness of urban poverty had long since pulverized whatever unifying traditions Appalachian or African-American families brought with them from the hollows or the Deep South. The Rez has its share of isolation and despair—alcoholics so poor they drank hairspray, children poisoned in their parents' crude meth lab—but urban despair looked more devastating and its victims more visible, if only because they were so many. Walking streets in the city's rougher neighborhoods in daylight, I glimpsed furtive eyes, hollow and dry as husks from last year's corn, while the soles of my shoes crunched over derelict cargo from the previous night: broken glass, empty packs of rolling papers, used condoms.

The clinic stood on a well-traveled street corner in a poor neighborhood, though not a frightening one. Our presence was welcomed by neighbors who looked out for the building after hours. Most local excitement happened while we were away. One Monday morning, as I stepped from my car in the parking lot, I caught the odor of wood smoke before noticing that much of the brick building on the far corner was now a burned-out shell. Clinic staff members who lived closest heard sirens and saw a lurid glow on Saturday night. Some drove by Sunday morning to make sure the clinic was unharmed, which it was. Others shared their surprise that the apartments hadn't burned down years before. We were grateful no one had been seriously hurt.

Daytime drama, when it visited the clinic, was less apocalyptic: addicts shouting in the waiting room, a gang assault victim stumbling through the front door, an elderly woman who lost consciousness while driving and plowed her car into a truck stopped at the intersection. I was among the first to attend to her while we waited for the ambulance to arrive, urging her to remain flat on the front seat and not move her left leg where an exposed, ragged edge of fractured tibia, slowly shedding drops of dark blood, jutted at an angle from her shin. Even as we heard sirens approaching, she stared into space with wide, frightened eyes and muttered, "Tell them to come quickly. Tell them to come quickly." When the EMTs arrived, I turned her over to their capable hands and readier equipment. One was already working on an IV before they closed the ambulance doors to drive away. I later learned she made it through that night, though not the next.

My clinic colleagues—doctors, nurses, social workers, and front desk staff—were dedicated professionals who chose to work among the inner-city poor rather than somewhere more comfortable and lucrative. I liked my patients, even those whose parents seemed forever angry or more certain than I what prescription their children needed for whatever ailed them. Children are sturdy creatures. They often get better despite what the pediatrician does. A maxim every student hears in medical school is *Primum non nocere*: "First, do no harm." The hard-won practical wisdom of medicine lies not so much in knowing what to do, but when, how, and to whom—and the greatest of these may well be when: when to lance the boil, when to prescribe medicine, when to consult the subspecialist or admit to the hospital. This wisdom entails, of course, knowing when *not* to act. When doctors fall for the "Politician's Fallacy":

A. Something must be done.

B. This is something.

C. Therefore, I must do this,

patients get hurt. I spent much of my time talking parents out of unnecessary antibiotics, cold remedies, or pain medications. But I was in the company of children, and that covered a multitude of sins.

An inner city clinic running on a shoestring budget expects its share of problems recruiting and retaining staff. Fine, hard-working doctors came and went, marginal ones avoided calling attention to themselves, and the executive director, who had once been a professional gambler, did everything necessary to keep the doors open and the lights on. A small nonprofit organization like the clinic can be lean and nimble in times of change and uncertainty, but much depends on personnel. If a key worker leaves, the right replacement may not be available in the organization and difficult to lure from the outside. The wrong person can be disastrous. There are, I've found, far worse things than an unfilled position. With leanness comes vulnerability.

As more experienced providers moved on, I took on more responsibility. Having worked for the Feds, I understood turnover, limits, and the need for flexibility. When I was asked to become medical director, I accepted the role as a necessary stopgap, insisting I was only *acting* medical director until a long-term successor could be found. I quickly learned two things: I could do the job, and I hated it. I wanted to care for kids, not patch schedule holes, review budgets, and chat with salesmen. I also had more weekend duty than ever before, with a sharp increase in parental phone calls at all hours. The clinic couldn't afford a phone triage service with on-call nurses fielding standard questions about diarrhea and colds and passing more complicated matters along to the on call physician. I found it impossible to stay pleasant, professional, and patient-centered while taking, at 2 am, the hundredth call of the weekend about the latest intestinal virus.

William Osler would not have approved. I lacked the stoic detachment he prized in a physician, the ability to face frustrations and failures with unshakeable calm. I wanted to be Osler's man, but I couldn't. My body betrayed my emotions. My mind would not keep its distance. I fumed. I stewed. Sometimes I even complained out loud.

Complaining about job satisfaction when most of my patients were struggling to pay the bills seemed rather rich—pun fully accounted for. I met with the executive director, who was sympathetic and promised to find a permanent medical director as soon as possible, but the only person with whom I truly shared my unhappiness was Jill. As in Tuba City, she wanted to see me smile again, to wake up in the morning with something other than resignation. Once again, she wanted her husband back.

A morning came when I left the house, climbed into the car, slid the key into the ignition and, with a long and weighty sigh, muttered, "How am I going to get through this day?" I could no longer deny I was at an impasse. I mustered enough strength to drive to work, see my patients, put out the administrative fires, and return home, but I'd clearly crossed a professional Rubicon. When Jill and I talked after dinner, the question was no longer *if* I should find another place to work, but how quickly. Somewhere I could see patients—preferably on the lower end of the economic ladder—and leave schedules and salesmen to someone else. Somewhere with a phone triage system, and less likely to colonize the time I hoped to spend with my family. Somewhere I might even stop talking about writing and embrace the discipline of wordcraft.

I left the inner city clinic in northern Kentucky soon after, moving to the Ohio side of the river to join a new storefront primary care office affiliated with the University of Cincinnati. It was what businesspeople call "a cold start," a brand new primary care office in a "medically underserved" neighborhood. The going was slow at the beginning, but word spread and patients came. The neighborhood was in transition: an aging first-tier suburb abandoned by wealthier residents for exurbs metastasizing ever farther from the city core. Lower middle class and working poor families took their places, folks less able to disguise the chaos of their lives with manners and money. I met families where both parents worked, but needed public assistance to feed their children. Teenaged girls with perfect hair visited repeatedly for pregnancy tests, brushing aside offers of contraception as "too much trouble." I only saw the boys with whom they traded sex for affection when they needed a physical exam for high school sports. The place and its people teetered on the rim of a social cliff. I felt ill-suited to the task of catching people before they ran over the edge.

* * * *

That same year, Jill and I traveled to Guatemala to adopt our daughter, Maria. With two "biological" sons already, we were open to other ways of welcoming children to our family. We worked through the long process of applications, home evaluations, classes, international documents, and fees. Then we waited. After weeks without word from the adoption agency, Jill received an agency call about a boy and girl—unrelated but suddenly available on the same day—in Guatemala. Unless we wanted both—a turn we weren't prepared for—we had to choose. Until then, we'd said that male or female didn't matter, but Jill made up our minds instantly, shouting, "I want a girl!" We named her Maria Judith, after my mother, Mary, and my godmother and favorite aunt, Judy.

The boys stayed at home with our Cincinnati babysitter while Jill and I flew south, landing in Guatemala City late on a spring-like November afternoon. As twilight blurred into blackness, we rode a taxi to the hotel, the route illumined with billboards and electric signs advertising North American fast food. The road ahead divided into lanes of headlights and taillights, with alarming jumbles of white and red at various intervals, darting and weaving without pattern. When we arrived at the hotel, our daughter was waiting for us in a sitting room next to the lobby, seated in her foster mother's lap, twirling her right foot in slow circles and smiling demurely at her many admirers. She wore her best clothes: a blue print baby outfit with red vest, and a white bow in her jet-black hair. Jill and I froze in the doorway, wordlessly watching, faces aglow, both of us instantly, totally, and irrevocably in love with a stranger we'd just met.

Maria, only nine months old, wasn't sure what to make of the new white faces thrust suddenly into her life. I blew soapsud bubbles to amuse her and Jill gave her a bottle when she grew hungry. We talked with the foster family and representatives from the adoption agency for over an hour. Her foster mother and sisters presented us with several baby dresses, some formula, and her favorite bottle, as well as a diary of our daughter's stay with their family. She'd clearly been doted on by her four foster sisters, who had changed her outfits several times daily, fed her as often as possible, and carried her in their arms throughout the day. There were "thank yous" and tears all around as the family departed. Maria looked crestfallen as we prepared for bed, but when the three of us awoke the next morning as early light flooded the spare, airy room, we were without question a family.

And so we became newly vulnerable. Just after breakfast, a Canadian couple arrived at the hotel, distraught and weeping, having just heard that the child they were there to adopt had been kidnapped. Many hours later, after a day of utter panic, they were reunited with their baby: the foster mother had secretly taken the child to another home in a bizarre—and unsuccessful—ploy to persuade the Canadians that she'd make an ideal nanny. When the kidnapping story unraveled late that night and the baby returned to the adoptive parents, there was, of course, no chance of that happening.

But there was an ugly context to the episode that made the long hours of uncertainty all the more sinister. With North Americans adopting Guatemalan children in increasing numbers late in the course of the country's thirty-six-year-long civil war, some locals, for political reasons or simply to keep outsiders away, spread tales of Americans flying children north and harvesting their organs for transplantation. No tangible evidence was presented to support these grisly claims, but the goal of these rumors was fear, not truth. There were more than enough believable stories of Americans operating outside the standard adoption process. There were also tales of Americans assaulted or jailed in rural villages, reportedly over poorly handled adoption inquiries, but these, too, were murky. Getting to the truth was difficult, perhaps impossible.

The adoption agency strongly advised couples to be vigilant while in Guatemala, avoid crowds, and limit the time they spent in public with their new child. We did as instructed, adding a macabre undercurrent to an otherwise joyful mission. All this was on our minds when we met the distraught Canadians. In the agony in their searching eyes, the catch in their voice as they spoke, we saw reflections of our own vulnerability. And we, having given our hearts to our daughter, painfully relearned the First Lesson of Parenthood. We were not in control.

Morning's sadness colored the remainder of the day. Sudden rain showers filled then fled an otherwise sunny sky. We busied ourselves with trips to the US Consulate, paperwork, and getting to know our daughter during long waits. On one such wait, I took a taxi to the *Mercado Central* while Jill and Maria napped in the security of the hotel. Sunlight, slanting though scattering rainclouds, revealed much the night had obscured: the chaotic elegance of five traffic lanes on a two lane highway, teenagers in fatigues pacing before government buildings with automatic weapons at the ready, the vibrant sadness of a people waiting to declare a long civil war officially over. The *Mercado* pulsed with life, but the shopkeepers' averting eyes betrayed a dark sadness. The indigenous stoicism I knew from living with the Navajo was not to be found, replaced here by world-weary Ladino *tristeza*. As I emerged from a shadowy row of stands piled with textiles, a young man purposefully approached and began a conversation in reasonably good English. We talked awhile, more in English than Spanish, and he offered to show me around the nearby plaza.

"What would you like to see?" he asked.

Not sure what he had in mind, but knowing the Metropolitan Cathedral was close at hand, I said "*la iglesia*," and off we went. As we walked together, however, his questions grew increasingly pointed and probing—Who was I? What did I do in the States? What was I doing in Guatemala? How long was I staying and where? My answers turned cagier, more opaque. The morning's events weighed on my mind. I was also well aware that the United States had played an unsavory role in the not-quite-ended civil war. I looked for ways to break off the expedition. We ended up sipping *café con leche* at a table in a small *tienda*, where my self-appointed tour guide insisted I give him my address in the States so he could visit me later. When polite attempts at deflection failed, I took a pen and wrote on a white paper napkin a fake last name and the address of my long-since abandoned medical school apartment in St. Louis, and said I had to meet someone soon. We stood up, said our *hastas*, and parted.

Heading back to the hotel in a taxi, I puzzled over what had just happened. I'd felt an introvert's distress over not knowing the rules the game, but there was more. I usually find encounters abroad intriguing, a chance to learn and practice the language, but I'd been unnerved at finding myself in over my head. For all I know, my Guatemalan guide may have been no more than excessively curious, but as his questions turned prying, I desperately wanted to be elsewhere, safe with my wife, our new daughter, our sons.

Back at the hotel, Jill sat in a sunny windowsill, reading alongside a napping Maria. I debated awakening the baby for an urgently needed hug, but stood at the open doorway instead, wordlessly watching my wife smile and our daughter sleep. They were safe, and I was with them. Later that afternoon, as we walked to the consulate to receive our final documents, I carried Maria in my arms with new vigilance, imagining potential threats in everyone we encountered. Guatemala is a beautiful, sad place, and I knew I would return, but just then I wanted to be elsewhere. I wanted to be home.

There were no unpleasant surprises or disasters for the remainder of our stay, though we were in no state to appreciate it. After finishing our official business, we went directly back to the hotel and quietly readied for the flight home next morning. Maria slept well—a fact Jill and I were able to verify as we slept fitfully, if at all. We awoke early and bleary-eyed, ate a quick breakfast, grabbed our luggage, and boarded a taxi to the airport. Our taxi driver smiled at the three of us and offered a soft *felicidades*, to which I rendered a weak *gracias*. The remainder of the drive was silent, our faces determined, our daughter all contentment. At the airport, I spied the Canadian couple, beaming as the pushed their baby in a stroller.

"You found her?" I asked excitedly.

"Yes," they shouted, and shared the events of the previous night: frantic calls to the agency and Guatemalan authorities; long taxi rides to false leads; the foster mother, sensing the plan wasn't going well, finally revealing her deception; and the nighttime recovery of their baby from a cardboard and sheet metal shack. The baby was fine, and the Canadians, having no interest in pressing kidnapping charges against a woman clearly desperate to leave the country, were content to refer matters to the adoption agency.

We shared our relief, offered congratulations, and parted with warm embraces and wishes for an uneventful return home. Jill and I joined the queue at the passport checkpoint. More accurately, we joined the fast-moving North Americans who were waved forward without an inspection of their documents. To our right snaked a long, stationary column of working class Guatemalans in what were likely their best clothes, suffering the conspicuous disregard of the official who would, they hoped, finally permit them to board a flight to somewhere else. Jill and I boarded our plane, remembering at the gate that we had first class seats, the only ones available when we booked our flight on short notice. Businessmen looked up from day-old *Wall Street Journals* and tumblers of whiskey, eyeing us suspiciously as we took our seats. But Maria, who remained quietly content as long as Jill held her, soon won them over with her smile. Jill sighed in relief when the plane lifted from the tarmac. Maria smiled, cooed, and slept most of the flight north, and when we touched down in the States, Jill turned to our daughter and said, "We're home."

* * * *

Returning home meant returning to work. After a brief paternity leave, I returned to the storefront clinic. While there, I re-entered the world of medical teaching as an attending. I began supervising nurse practitioner students in the office and pediatric residents in the outpatient clinic at Cincinnati Children's Hospital. Some needed habits came easily: the back and forth of question and answer, the necessary restraint to permit learners to show what they know, and the insight to gauge what they're ready for more. The challenge, I found, is to bring the student to a place of appropriate discomfort, allowing her to work at the frontiers of her abilities, while making clear I'll stop her before she does something dangerous.

For introverts, teaching requires a persona, a role one assumes. It's an effort on my part to remain present in a group. Personae—roles taken on in certain situations—afford breathing room, a social place where I know some of the rules, where I can be less anxious about how to behave, what to say next. "Teacher" was a role I lived into. In time, teaching claimed a growing part of my workweek. I moved from the storefront clinic to a teaching clinic near the hospital, still seeing my own patients while carving out time to supervise residents in the office and on hospital wards.

Even as I learned new lessons and acquired new skills, a hollowness lingered in my daily life that sapped what might have been unadulterated satisfaction. I taught residents habits that served me well, but to what end? No matter how I tried to greet each patient with the special delight of a parent, I lost my way in the depths of cold and flu season. I knew from experience the powerful, protective love of a parent for a child, but the day-long pageant of snot, wheezing, and watery diarrhea made me long for June, when kids are generally healthy and elsewhere. In the busiest of times, the persona of teacher or doctor became a tight-fitting mask, protective and confining. I wore it faithfully while pushing through a crowded schedule, until my face conformed to it rather than the other way round. Duty conquered delight.

Jill arrived at a similar impasse, confident in her skills but desiring new challenges. Never fully comfortable in the operating room, she pondered opportunities in public health, perhaps returning to school for a public health degree. We talked many times, asking each other, "What's next?" while reflecting on the changes we'd put us and our children through. In little more than five years, we had moved across the country, found new jobs, added a third child, and turned our lives around in search of a proper balance of pursuits, a place where all our affections—professional, personal, and family—fell happily together. We were closer to that goal, but what balance we had achieved seemed precarious at best. A seemingly minor change, like becoming medical director, might topple everything. We could do nothing and assume the best, or we could take some pre-emptive action. At the time, the answer seemed clear. We were ready for something more. We only had to decide what it would be.

Chapter Nine

Baltimore Interlude:
Scenes From a Year Away

Cincinnati, Ohio/Baltimore, Maryland

Leaving

"YOU ARE COMING BACK?" Rhonda asked, turning at last to face me. Who could blame her for being particular, for wanting to be sure? Her delight in Khalil, the infant she had just set on the examining table, was infectious. Rhonda, wrapped in Guinea brocade of orange, red, and black, was Khalil's adoptive mother, and I—an adoptive parent myself—served as pediatrician and biggest fan. Mother and child transformed the gray office walls, vivid assurance there was more to pediatrics than diarrhea and ear infections. Gray summed up what the practice had become—not always, but often. My routine had turned stale. Staff meetings, the intractable bureaucracy of a large hospital system, the nonsense of medical insurance and referrals: all weighed on me, fueling the sense that I was stuck.

Rhonda asked because I'd recently mailed my patients a letter with news that I planned to leave Cincinnati for a year. My family was temporarily relocating to Baltimore, Jill's hometown, where she'd study for a Master's Degree in Public Health at Johns Hopkins. I hoped that was all I needed to say, but Rhonda knew this was about more than meeting my wife's career needs. I love kids, and couldn't think of another specialty that would have held my interest even this long. Still, I had grave doubts about my future in a profession that had, to my surprise, ceased to delight. Maybe it was a passing phase. Maybe it was the turning point to a second career. Telling families that I wasn't sure I wanted to be a doctor any more seemed rather cold, and then I'd have to explain much more than I cared to. How much simpler to say it was my duty to go, that I wasn't abandoning anyone, that I'd be back in a year?

"That's the plan," I said, smiling at the precision of my ambiguity. Undeterred, Rhonda, her hand drifting over to touch Khalil's shoulder, trained her eyes on mine as she leaned slightly forward, her brow furrowed, wordlessly pressing me to say more.

I continued, "You've heard me say before that I've given up predicting the future, but we're certainly not planning on staying in Baltimore longer than we have to."

"Will you work there?"

"I get to be Dad. And I get to write."

"Oh yes," she said, "I remember you said you liked to write." She retreated a moment, as if considering whether to pursue an unpromising line of questioning, familiar as she was with my talent for evasion. When asked what I did with the weekday I wasn't in the office, I sometimes mentioned writing, but usually just replied, "I'm a much happier guy when I'm not in one place all the time."

Realizing she'd gain little through frontal assault, Rhonda entertained light chatter about Baltimore, in-laws, and the surprises of life, and I, suddenly a raconteur, grew eloquent, expansive, yet doggedly unrevealing. Khalil needed no shots, no blood tests or referrals that day, and the rest of my schedule was laden with sullen adolescents and babies rank with the latest gastrointestinal virus. Each one required care, concern, and all my attention, but for now, I wanted to spend time with people who left me feeling lighter than when we'd begun. We talked awhile.

Khalil whimpered, bored by his audience's inattention. Rhonda took him into her arms. I helped gather scattered bottles, stuffed animals, and two hefty appointment books into the blue satchel that always accompanied him. We walked together to the front desk to check out. At Khalil's next visit, he'd see a new pediatrician in the office, one Rhonda had met only that morning. I leaned toward the computer screen as the receptionist scheduled the appointment, verifying details. I wanted to take care of my friends. At the elevator, I gave Rhonda a hug and wondered, as I turned away, what had gone awry in my career as a doctor. The elevator doors closed, and I walked back to the examining rooms, stopping to frown at the afternoon appointment schedule.

Apart

The family the boys and I were housesitting for had lost the front door key years ago. Definitive exits went through the kitchen, taking care not to set the button lock, which likewise had no key. We went through the ritual each time: twisting the knob to make sure it rotated freely, closing the door carefully behind, finding the one useful key—mixed in with those of our own house, now rented for the year—and firmly grabbing the outer knob while turning the key in the deadbolt that grudgingly creaked home. Then the struggle of getting the boys in the car, making sure they'd brought everything for the pool, the park, or wherever we were heading that moment.

Days pulsed with improvised rhythms. Work no longer called the tune. Jill and Maria were already in Baltimore. Jill's parents baby-sat our daughter while Jill went to class. The boys remained with me in Cincinnati until swim season was over. Both Peter and Will expected to make the swim finals. Both were determined to play as much and as often as possible with friends they'd soon have to do without for nearly a year. The tenants moved into our old house on Fourth of July weekend, we evacuated to the home of friends who were spending the summer in Spain.

It's difficult for me to fall asleep, lying alone in someone else's bed. After reading the boys their stories (Will, at eleven, still insisted on a chapter at bedtime and I was too fond of words to deny him) and turning out the lights in borrowed bedrooms, my eyes dulled with the filmy hollowness of one displaced. I toured the rooms, aimlessly searching through another man's books, drinking another man's beer. The beer I'd replace. The books I envied.

In the dim light, I flipped through the notebooks the boys were keeping for their mother, diaries from which they could reconstruct their time apart. Seven-year-old Peter adopted a telegraphic style: "Had fun. Swam a lot today. Miss you." Will was more expansive, if similarly unrevealing, his prose littered with creative misspelling. Perhaps having a father who wrote for fun—or was it necessity?—made keeping a diary a chore. I was glad they made the effort. In contrast, I put precious little on paper, though there was time enough to read.

My year away from doctoring barely begun, I already felt pressure to achieve, to earn my idleness. I stared into middle distance, focusing on something suddenly irretrievable, like an actor groping for a forgotten line. The house hushed around me. Sagging bookshelves sat in judgment. I jerked my head toward a movement at the window and saw the cat pawing the glass. I walked to the door, opened it, and lured her inside. She followed me—at a distance—into the basement, where I filled her bowls with food and water. Turning off the lights again, I silently cataloged the life in this borrowed house. The cat was already eating, gently tipping the bowl in the darkness. An angelfish floated serenely among neon tetras in the murmuring kitchen aquarium. Upstairs, a turtle surveyed his glass-walled world.

I looked in on my sleeping boys, watching the tidal motion of their chests, faintly visible in the light of a single hallway lamp. I turned away slowly, headed back down to the living room. I felt too tired to read. Perhaps tonight I'd watch a movie. When it was over, it would be time to sleep.

Together

In Baltimore, together as a family again, Jill and I celebrated, packing up the car for a family camping trip to Assateague Island, on the Atlantic coast. We drove to the beach for our first ocean view of the trip, then went in search of a campsite. Amid the usual family chaos, we all seemed to be having a good time. But when wild horses ran through the nearly empty campground, Maria leapt to the safety of a picnic table. Making up in assertiveness what she lacked in height, four-year-old Maria took care of herself. Jill had explained to the children about the ponies of Assateague, how as a girl she had dreamed of buying one from the annual roundup on neighboring Chincoteague, and how she and I, years later, laughed at the signs throughout the National Seashore, warning "Wild ponies kick and bite." Jill imagined the Park Service overrun with litigation-shy killjoys bent on ruining her childhood memories of Marguerite Henry's *Misty of Chincoteague* and *Stormy, Misty's Foal*. On the other hand, Maria, for all her love of cuteness and fuzz, had sufficient reason to fear large, charging, unpredictable beasts. Afterward, ferociously gripping her mother's neck, she confessed, "I was a little afraid, because I didn't know where they were going." Jill, suddenly the mother bear, cursed the horses and clutched her daughter to her chest.

Few campers stayed on Assateague that August. Insect swarms, denser than usual after recent summer downpours, drove overnighters away. Campsites close to the beach, where a steady wind kept the voracious mosquitoes and black flies at bay, were easy to find. Horses were infrequent visitors. They quickly moved on if no one defied park rules and fed them. We planned to camp for two nights, celebrating the boys' safe arrival on the

East Coast, but gray-black clouds stretched in a solid, roiling mass from mainland to the easternmost horizon of the leaden sea.

Not easily discouraged, we scouted for a likely campsite with level sand and no standing water or horse manure. While we set up our tent, Maria remained alert for horses as her brothers slapped at mosquitoes and obsessed over DEET, applying thick layers of insect repellant so frequently I finally took the bottle and hid it in the car. For dinner, we ate spaghetti ladled from a pot on the Coleman stove. Citronella candles flickered on the table like votive lamps. Afterwards, we crawled into our tents in the cloud-covered early twilight, zipping the insect netting tight while I inspected the rain fly. The ritual, however comforting, later proved useless, overmatched by the coming deluge. That night, drops gathered into rivulets along waterproofed seams as rain cascaded from the fly, lines snapped and sagged with each slap of the wind, and bodies nudged together at the tent's center, away from the billowing walls. In the sickly pallor of a gray and windy morning, Jill and I, who hadn't slept well, surveyed the damp sleeping bags and dripping clothes and knew we'd spend the coming night in a hotel. This was, after all, our first weekend back together.

Both

The wind rose, heavy with the scent of more rain, rustling the pages of the book on the bench beside me. I reached for it, pressing the cover down. The soccer field was too far from home for the boys to walk. Rather than driving the round trip twice, I stayed though each practice, sitting in the bleachers with a book. Not that I got much reading done. Whoever practiced that evening wanted to be watched, though Will grew indignant if my parental interest was too obvious. I was already learning the subtle art of cloaking attention with feigned detachment. The other kids—the ones not scheduled for practice that evening—rarely entertained themselves, so they came along whenever Jill had homework, which became every night. Early in the year, she postponed studying until the kids were in bed. She'd spent the entire day away from the kids she loved, and she needed time to play with them again. "Take your book to practice," she said, "I'll keep the others with me." But as schoolwork accumulated, she needed time in the evenings to study and write. On her writing nights, I took all three children. This was a father's privilege; why wasn't I grateful? The four-year-old played on the small playground near the practice fields and the eight-year-old had always been a loner, but the eleven-year-old needed action. If Will had no friends along for the ride, I gave up watching, put down the book, and traded shots on goal or tossed a baseball with him. At such times, I sometimes felt put upon, and that, in turn, made me feel ashamed.

I knew mothers who spend every waking moment with their children and never complained. At least not to me. Single mothers bring their children to me for pediatric care, and several chose solo parenthood through adoption or other, less conventional, arrangements. Sure, they had their troubles, and I was glad to listen to them. I reassured each one of them that they were doing well, that they should be proud of what they were doing. Some even adopted again, and I was happy for them, however much it appeared to me a triumph of hope over experience.

"What's with these people?" I wondered, fully aware that it was the wrong question. This was my year to learn the joys of being a full-time dad. I could look at my taxi service duty as time away from writing to enjoy my children—it was my choice. For the month of August, there were four trips a week to the soccer fields, two evenings for each boy. Maria, ever sensitive to others' needs, was happy for her brothers but crushed that our new neighborhood, unlike the one we'd left in Cincinnati, had no soccer teams for four-year-old girls. To make it up, we planned to enroll her in gymnastics that fall.

I started to add up the hours of sports-related driving ahead. Wrong way to look at it, I decided. How about the friends the kids will make this way? Soccer teams were connected to school, so this was the perfect introduction to a new group of kids they'd be spending time with in the year ahead. That would mean play dates and more driving. Ugh. Had I known that, by the time regulation soccer gave way to indoor soccer, which finally ended in early spring, each boy would play nearly forty games, I might have rethought the entire year.

Morning

6:15 am.

The radio. NPR. *Morning Edition.*

Blind stabs at the snooze button.

Silence.

6:22

Nina Totenberg from the Supreme Court.

Same response.

Silence.

6:29

NPR's corporate underwriters.

Local weather.

Garrison Kiellor and the *Writer's Almanac*. The day's poem. The tossing back of bedcovers. The creaking of sleep-stiffened joints.

Thus armed, we rise, heading for the bathroom. Showering together, Jill and I share minutes awake and undisturbed. We embrace under a rush of hot water, lather snaking down wet skin, each choosing an emotional shield for a day apart. She thinks of friends at school and how she'll play with the children when she returns that evening. I imagine writing in the silence of an empty house.

We dry off in warm mist. I wrap a towel around my waist and awaken the boys. Neither takes the news well. Odd, how on weekend mornings they rise early, without prodding and moaning. Maria, hearing the house come alive, calls from her bedroom, demanding hot chocolate. I humor her into saying, "Please." I stir chocolate into microwaved milk and wonder if my children are past all hope of civility. Childhood cuteness must be a necessary biological adaptation, deterring parents from clobbering offspring who so richly deserve it.

With encouragement, Maria mutters "thank you" when handed the cup. Will is clattering out the front door, returning in moments with the morning paper, tearing through the sheaf for the sports section, leaving the rest scattered on the table like hulls of shucked corn. Peter says he's cold and sits sullenly on the living room chair, pulling a woolen blanket over the short sleeve shirt he's chosen to wear today. Maria wants help picking out her clothes, then says she'll do it herself. This is not a family of morning people.

Jill will take the early bus this morning. She slurps yogurt and Vitamin C while gathering her papers for the day. Though she feels the burden of her work, it's a good week. She feels she's on to something now, that she hasn't needlessly uprooted her family. She loves her children, still can't entirely shake the guilt of not staying at home with them, but knows she'd swiftly lose her mind doing that. School, unlike work or family, offers targets to work for. No one ever gives her an "A" for spending time with her children.

For me, culpability comes from not working. I felt it when I went to a part-time schedule, hairs rising on my neck like a dog guarding his turf whenever asked where I spent my "free days." I feel it more intensely now, particularly when Jill's ready to leave, while I'm still slipping on my jeans, thankful I don't need to dress up, that I can go without a tie for months and never feel underdressed. I hurry to kiss Jill at the back door before she goes.

Children slither to the table. Will, engrossed in baseball statistics, needs three reminders to eat his breakfast. Peter finishes his Fruit Loops in seconds, managing for once to spill less than half the bowl. Maria, having chosen petulance as this morning's attitude, rejects all the boxes of cereal. Will, still uninterested in eating, offers to make her toast. As the idea doesn't come from Dad, she agrees.

I warn the children of imminent departure. No one responds. I offer incentives, remembering not to call them threats. Glacial activity ensues. Incentives escalate until everyone is out the door. I herd them to the car, lowering my voice so as not to alarm the neighbors. Seat belts are buckled, last minute arguments arbitrated. The children launch a new campaign: they want the radio on to their favorite station, "the best mix of the '80s, '90s, and today." I back out from the carport, my passengers sedated by morning radio chatter.

Another day.

Noon

Never is the need to dust above the refrigerator so urgent as when I sit down to write. Never does my moustache so need trimming as when I start a new paragraph. "Now it's time to write," I tell myself, "Write, damn it."

Is an audience required for performance anxiety? Does the dog count? Blondie, the Rez dog, sprawls at the far end of the room, eyeing me for hints of activity, preliminaries to a walk. Is there a human in the audience? Jill will ask later if I got any work done today. I used to be frustrated when she read my work and merely said, "That's good." Now I'm peeved by her targeted criticisms, most of them disturbingly right. Couldn't she find a judicious middle ground, something like, "I think if you flesh out these descriptive passages, you'd raise the entire work from Pulitzer quality to Nobel?"

Food. A legitimate interruption. I must eat to keep glucose streaming to my brain. Graze cupboards. Visit the refrigerator. Assess the leftovers.

Coffee. Who can write without caffeine? Boil water. Grind the beans. Search for a can of evaporated milk; there's no cream to be had. Get another cup. Bathroom break.

Now I'm thirsty again, having already peed off a liter. Find something without caffeine, preferably without calories. Too many snacks for one morning.

Who will care, who will even know if I don't write? My advisor, for one. I'm doing independent study in writing Johns Hopkins, paying someone to keep me honest. Without accountability, temptations to dither smother all else like kudzu on a neglected hillside. I appreciate having someone to send material to, someone I can trust to say, "This is terrible," without worrying about the effect on the relationship. I like deadlines. They keep me on track. For some people, the lure of money pales in comparison to the power of guilt and shame. As long as cash is available, I indulge myself by claiming that money management is beyond my understanding. Guilt and shame— that I get. They've been the backbone of medical education for decades. All the incentive I need comes packaged as promises and deadlines. Failure is no longer acceptable if someone will know. I sit, suppressing the image of dishes in the sink yet unwashed from breakfast. I'll stay at the keyboard now, my motivation clear.

It's time to write.

Write, damn it.

Night

Dusk comes quickly when daylight savings ends. By the time I drive the kids back from school and start dinner, the eastern horizon, visible through the window above the kitchen sink, turns cold and blue. Already four months into our adventure, and my hopes of literary accomplishment, of greatness begun, scatter like globs of oil in the dishwater before me. I blame family responsibilities, even as I skillfully murder each gift hour with practiced want of purpose. I have a point on Wednesdays, a day spent volunteering in Peter's class, shopping for groceries, a week of errands packed into twenty-four hours. The rest of the week, though, the argument falls flat.

Pots mutter on the stove, while I rinse the congealed crust of breakfast from neglected bowls. I set them carefully, one to a slot, in the drying rack that I'll empty and fill two or three more times before I go to bed tonight. When asked once by a friend—a woman—if I did all the housework while Jill went to school, I surprised her with the vehemence of my denial. I'd read somewhere that American men consistently overestimate their contribution to the family, that the time difference spent in housework between men who say they share chores and those who say they don't is a mere six minutes. Despite her academic demands, Jill enjoys cooking and often does laundry. I take out the trash but never clean the bathroom. This year, I'm not even paying the bills.

From her bedroom, Maria calls, asking me to read her a book. I throttle a sigh. We meet in the living room and sit together on the couch. She brings a picture book about a bear family, part of a series of stories I'm familiar with. Like all the others, this one ends with the blustery buffoon of a father rescued from near disaster by his long-suffering children and forgiving wife. Maria, who only took this book out of the library yesterday, knows it by heart, as if she'd written it herself. She asks me to read it once again. "No," I says. "I have to finish making dinner. Mommy will be home soon."

"I want Mommy now," she says. I stand, listening for the back door, the creaking of which announces Jill's arrival. Nothing.

"Not long. Not long, Maria," I say, hoping she finds comfort in my vagueness. I turn to face her and find her already spread out on the couch, head against a pillow.

"Don't fall asleep, yet, Maria. We're going to eat soon." I almost say, "As soon as Mommy gets here," but quit before making that blunder. She infers it anyway.

"Go away," Maria says, her temper rising, her face a hybrid of grimace and pout.

Returning to the kitchen, I check the calendar to see whose week it is to set the table. Peter. He won't be happy about it. He never is. I choose not to bother him yet. I'll call in ten minutes. Why disturb him when he's playing quietly? I start water for the pasta, add salt, rinse lettuce for a salad. This year, I remind myself, there are no patients in distress, no nightly barrage of phone calls. Here's the freedom I've coveted. The entire family will be together tonight, uninterrupted, unrushed.

I hope they eat what I'm making.

Doctor

The operating room complex at the hospital in Tuba City looks unchanged. I had reason to be here often enough when we called the Navajo Rez home, and now I'm back for a short stay, filling in for one of the staff pediatricians. I'm trying to remember the name of the surgical assistant when she turns and gasps, "What are you doing here?"

Navajo inflections grace her speech, consonants clipped short, vowels cradled near the tongue's root. She rises from the supply cupboard she's been searching, looking genuinely pleased to see me, if a bit startled. I start to reach for a Navajo handclasp and a soft, "*Yáʼátʼééh,*" then think better of it, and hug her instead.

She laughs readily, her short, ample frame rumbling. She looks me over, reassuring herself this familiar face is no illusion, then asks, "You here to stay?"

Color rises in my sun-starved cheeks. "No, I'm just here three weeks. Dr. Moul's father is sick, and he needed some time off, so I'm filling in."

"Where are you living now?"

"We're spending a year in Baltimore while Jill goes back to school."

"Izzit?" In my five years on the Reservation, I never quite understood what that opaque local expression meant. Something to do with mild surprise. Another Navajo-ism *bilagáanas* don't get. I nod blankly.

There's much more I don't understand. Why, for instance, had I left the desert at all, more than six years ago?

Now I was back, feeling like a has-been nightclub singer making a comeback stab with a limited engagement off the Vegas Strip. I've stumbled into a cliché: former headliner drifts into a fantasy past. The hospital changed little in my absence. It's easy to imagine I've awakened from a vivid dream and found myself back home.

Standing in surgical scrubs outside the operating room, waiting for the anesthetist to start an epidural before the Caesarian section begins, I recount the events leading to this return. Dr. Moul had mentioned his father's illness before, but hadn't told me how advanced it was. By December, he was in precipitous decline, and Dr. Moul, knowing where he was needed, took himself out of the January schedule. That's when the other pediatricians made the call to Baltimore and, for the first time since my relocation back east, I could help them out. Of course, it worked both ways. After six months of squandering our savings, my family could use the income. It was time I made some money and recaptured a sense of worth.

Nonetheless, it frightened me to think how much could happen in three weeks, especially in a hospital. I'd never been entirely confident of my skills, despite my genuine credentials, the imposing initials after my name, and the polite encouragement of friends. Now, while I fret over all I'd forgotten in six years away from hospital medicine, I'm finding out how much is still there, waiting to be used. Even the finer skills, like starting IVs in an infant's threadlike veins, remained in muscular memory, returning with astonishing thoroughness and detail, more like remembering a well-rehearsed piano sonata than riding a bike. There was something fun in being a doctor, after all. "I could do this again," I thought.

Could I? Hadn't I spent recent years wondering how to escape? What about all those promises I'd made to himself about finding time to write, to do what made me happy instead of doing my duty. But didn't this—doctoring for people who thought, despite my many doubts, that I was rather good at it—make me happy, in its own way? Was all that literary stuff a false scent, or was the Teutonic duty-monster awakening within, whispering I was nothing if not the family's breadwinner and a tireless servant of the suffering and needy?

"The trouble is," I realize, "there's no obvious wrong here. Once again, it's not a question of bad and good, but a choice between different goods and whether one can be sustained without the other."

I just then remember where I am, and find the surgical assistant, whose name I still can't recall (Esther? Shirley?) staring at me as though I've lost my mind. Perhaps I have. I make small talk, which has never been my strong suit. Fortunately, she knows who I am, asks about Jill and the kids: questions for which I have a script of ready answers.

At last the circulating nurse leans through the doorway and says, "Pardon me, but we're getting ready to have a baby in here."

I blush, recalling not only precisely where I am, but also why I'm wanted. I say a quick, "Nice talking to you," to the surgical assistant, pull on my mask, and step into the OR, camouflaging embarrassment with purposeful activity. The obstetrician is already drawing her scalpel across the draped, iodine-stained globe of maternal flesh. Behind the drape, the anesthetist whispers reassurances to Mom. My own place, in the heat of the neonatal resuscitation table, stands empty, oxygen hissing from an anesthesia bag hanging like a limp snake ready to be skinned. I reexamine the instruments one by one, the same tools I carefully checked fifteen minutes ago. I know what I'm supposed to do. We're getting ready to have a baby.

Patient

Later, when she returned from the Baltimore hospital, Jill said a phone ringing at 3 a.m. either means a wrong number or very bad news. I'm the lighter sleeper, so I'd risen to answer the call this morning, and when I stayed on the kitchen phone speaking in short, widely-spaced sentences, Jill guessed, still huddled in the dissipating warmth of her bed, that it wasn't a wrong number. When I brought the phone to her, she knew.

My mother-in-law apologized for bothering us with news of Jill's father's heart attack. Bill wasn't the sort for heart troubles. At seventy-five, he'd had white hair for four decades, camouflaging any aging he'd gotten around to. Except for increasing complaints about slowing down, about his body not fulfilling his intentions, one might have imagined him frozen in indeterminate middle age. Jealous of his autonomy, quick to argue but readier to schmooze and charm, he'd awakened his wife that night to say he felt ill, that she needed to drive him to the Emergency Room, and that she was to tell no one.

He had the courtesy to delay the actual heart attack until he was on hospital monitors. A dozen white coats converged on him in seconds, shouting orders, starting IVs, pushing medications. That's when Jill's mother called and Jill said, without being asked, "I'll be right in." When Jill arrived, once the ruckus had died down, Bill, predictably, turned to his wife and said, "I told you not to call anybody."

"I'm not here for you," Jill said, assuming his bravado, "I'm here for her." She reached across the bed for her mother, who took her hand.

Before we moved, Jill promised that a year in Baltimore would, if nothing else, leave me as annoyed with her family's quirkiness as she was with mine. Her side, which regularly tested the health of any relationship with argument, speculation, and complaint, lost its collective tongue when one of their own became vulnerable. Despite the seriousness of Bill's condition, there were few expressions of tenderness. Going to his cardiac catheterization the next day, Jill's Dad barked out orders for his funeral. If he had to go down, he'd go in charge.

Tests revealed healthy heart muscle tenuously supplied by obstructed arteries, leaving no choice but surgery. The following day (Good Friday, by coincidence), Jill spent twenty hours at the hospital, waiting with her mother—whose name was Zenia, though everyone called her Zee—through the endless pre-op rituals, the surgery itself, and Bill's return to the CICU. Zee, who only the week before had unexpectedly blurted out, "You're going to miss me when you go back to Cincinnati," talked of everything but the matter at hand. At last, exhausted but reassured by the surgeon that her husband was doing well, she faced her daughter and said, "Thank you for coming. I needed someone here. Now I'm going home."

Jill stayed, talking with her brother, Mark, about being a parent to one generation while still a child of another, of seeing one's father seriously ill, potentially near death. Struggling with the language of vulnerability, they reminisced into the night, stepping out for a drink at a nearby bar while their father slept. There was a great deal to remember, to learn. Jill called me to check how the kids were doing, grateful we were all in town when this happened.

I listened, reassured, agreed, while I silently wondered how things would have played out had we been working in Cincinnati? Jill would have had to clear her schedule and make emergency travel plans. I wouldn't have had the luxury of pushing my writing aside to solo the kids through Easter vacation from school. Surely there was material in this latest trial, something I could turn into an essay, a story. Nothing reveals character so thoroughly as a close encounter with mortality. This was an opportunity to learn. All I needed to do was pay attention. Yet, even as I rose to the occasion, the kids clamoring about me, my thoughts turned inward, spiraling into a tailspin of ugly introspection.

As Jill's shaken family reckoned with its medical and emotional history, I pondered mine: German, reticent, pathologically cerebral, with a pervasive history of depression. I'd grown up among garden-variety melancholics: no suicides, no life-saving shock therapy, no recovered memories of unspeakable and unverifiable abuse; just chronic, low-grade dissatisfaction descending periodically into cycles of crippling self-recrimination. I remembered Randy, a visiting professor I'd worked with some years before, who insisted male depression was the father's fault, passed from generation to generation like Original Sin. Randy pressed pop psychology books on me with the prim ferocity of a door-to-door missionary. I dutifully read the first, finding it full of intriguing theories but disappointingly thin on substance. As attractively Oedipal as Randy's theory was—claiming victimhood for myself while tossing all the blame on Dad—I couldn't buy it. My father was, if anything, less flawed, more loving than I. Yet the doubts sown by Randy's psychoevangelism still gnawed, particularly now, while I struggled to be attentive father, comforting husband, and dutiful son-in-law all at once. The real and constant neediness of my children made painfully clear to me what role was my weakest.

Was I passing depression on to my children simply by being their father, infecting them through genetics or a grim psychodynamic legacy? More than a year ago, at Jill's urging, I reluctantly asked my doctor for medication, pills to purge melancholy. Life was better when serotonin lingered in my synapses, but was I merely covering up, treating the symptom and missing the disease? Psychiatry, I knew, was too rudimentary a science to answer that. It came down to belief, the rival religions of Freud and Jung, their squabbling descendants, and the medical modelers now in ascendancy. What was I to do?

For days I scourged himself, trying to think through my funk the way I, as a boy, scratched at poison ivy. The itch worsened; the blisters spread. Then, as if suddenly doused in Calamine, I stopped, unresolved questions pushed aside while I dealt with matters at hand. However inconvenient, my family needed attention. I never quite understood how it happened, but I was a father, connected to three children and their mother in ways not entirely of my choosing. Psychology, with its delusions of the imperial self, had little to say about it. Being a father wasn't something I could choose to put on the "to do" list each morning. "Dad" was one of my names.

In the darkness of the bedroom, I glanced at the phone, wondering if I should call Jill again to see how Bill was doing and find out when she might come home. I heard a familiar sound in the hallway, the quick steps of Maria heading to the bathroom. I listened to the tiny stream against the porcelain, the rustle of underclothes, the purposeful tugging at the toilet handle, the rush of water. Her face, brown and beautiful, appeared at the doorway.

"Is Mommy home yet, Daddy?"

"No, sweetheart. She's still at the hospital with Grandpa."

"Daddy. I'm thirsty. Can you get me a drink?"

I stifled a rising sigh and willed myself to feel the incredible gift in this moment.

"Sure, sweetheart."

Returning

We lay in bed together, husband and wife, side by side, reading silently. I held a copy of *How We Die*, hoping to take my mind off the day's frustrations. Jill glanced through the comics I dutifully set at her bedside table each evening. She was once again cross at my reluctance to talk. Just last night, I'd held Jill as she wept over the mistakes of the year, how she'd have taken different courses and worked with different professors had she known her job back in Cincinnati would vanish, casualty to a change in leadership in her division. Why couldn't I return the favor and complain while she comforted me?

Men.

It was already her last week of class, with only a paper and a group presentation between her and graduation. She still hadn't figured out what to do with a new set of initials appended to her name. We planned to return to Cincinnati, where we still owned a house surrounded by good friends, the kids were enrolled in schools they liked, and I, at least, still had a job, but we hadn't begun to pack. Jill was our strategist, the one to organize the grand projects, yet her mind was on other things. She'd have to cast a wider net for the year ahead, and we'd both begun thinking about places we might live besides Cincinnati. Perhaps even Baltimore.

Knowing how much Jill had on her mind already, I didn't confess my worries about money. She balanced the books while reassuring me that running up credit card debt was the American Way. Yet it went against the grain for me to shake off millennia of German frugality. Actually, I lost those habits quite easily, but never escaped the attendant anxiety. Worry was my preferred means of controlling the universe.

But there was liberation in reframing the question. Most of this year, I'd worried how to reenter the medical world back in Cincinnati, whether my adventure as father and writer would be put aside, written about later in the interstices of an office schedule. This new twist—Jill not having a job to return to—felt strangely like an expansion, as if someone removed a wall of painted scrim to reveal an enormous, unguessed-at stage set behind. I'd be back in medicine again soon—we needed the money—but the thought itself no longer carried claustrophobic dread. We'd think of something to do.

Turning pages, our hands touched, our fingers interlocking until I pulled away to mark my page and set the book on the bedside table. Jill dropped the comics. She turned toward my spreading arms, our bodies seeking familiar forms, her left thigh on my hip, her head against my shoulder.

We stayed that way, entwined silent, for several minutes. The dog wheezed at the bedside. Peter, turning in his sleep, thumped against the wall of the next room.

With a barely audible sigh, Jill spoke: "We have a lot to do."

And just before I reached to turn off the light, I said, "Yes, we do."

Chapter Ten

Khalil

Cincinnati, Ohio

"So you came back," Rhonda says as I enter the room. She doesn't sound shocked or excited. She sounds pleased: her words as always, spoken with warmth and quiet elegance. Rhonda's a wise woman. She's got style.

Her son brought us together. Rhonda and her husband, Abe, were Khalil's first and only foster parents. I've known them since his arrival in their home. Khalil's birth mother had a long list of problems and no prenatal care. She came to the hospital in labor, testing positive for cocaine. Hamilton County Social Services soon placed the newborn in foster care. I've heard nothing of Khalil's birth mother since. Rhonda and Abe had taken in children before, but they quickly realized that Khalil, however unpromising his start, was undefeatable. From the first time Rhonda and Abe placed this new child, smiling and wriggling, on my exam table, I understood, too: pay attention; here is a most special person.

"This one stays," Abe said to Rhonda one day, and Khalil stayed, part of their family forever. That was before they realized how complicated Khalil's medical care would become, but that, I'm certain, wouldn't have changed a thing.

The Khalil I've come to see today, the Khalil whose mother is glad I've returned, is not yet three, wide-eyed at a world full of promise and adventure, undaunted by encounters with hospitals and specialists. His narrow face shines liked polished mahogany, his eyes, his guileless grin fill the room

with light. No matter how dark my days in medicine get, I can find my way
with Khalil's smile.

I'm a pediatrician. I like almost all my patients. But Khalil is my
favorite patient. Ever. When he calls my name from the office hallway, I
smile. When he tosses his locks and grins at my wry, impossible questions, I
can't help but laugh. I've phoned his family on the slimmest medical excuse
just to get another dose of Khalil. When I mention our mutual patient to
Khalil's gastroenterologist, Dr. Kaul, it's like sharing a favorite joke with an
old friend. Dr. Kaul, stops, smiles, chuckles in his rich baritone and says,
"Ah yes, Khalil . . ." Like me, he's seen Khalil in pain, crestfallen at another
hospital admission, anxious over one more unpleasant procedure. Like me,
he marvels at the boy's resilience, at Abe and Rhonda's burning love. Khalil's
medical conditions are complex and occasionally baffling, his outpatient
chart uncommonly thick, but when I talk with specialists and consultants
who've met him, they don't consult their notes. They don't have to. No one
with half a heart forgets Khalil.

That I'm still a doctor is, in part, thanks to him. Doctoring, for all its privilege and wonder, wears me down. I stay with it, but at a cost visible only to
those who know me best: my wife, my children, me. Perhaps that's what
comes of being an introvert in a people-focused profession. There are moments: a toddler careening into my open arms, the exhausted bliss of new
parents, Honduran schoolgirls burying smiles in the palms of their hands.
They sustain me through the weary parade of winter coughs and wheezes, of
preteens with sexually transmitted infections, of troubling judgments about
a parent's care, or malice, or both. If I didn't love children, didn't speak to
them more comfortably, more authentically than I talk to adults, I would
have drifted into some other line of work years ago. I don't know what I'll
do when my knees grow stiff, when I can't crouch, see eye to eye with my
patients, lie down on the floor and play.

Our family's interlude in Baltimore, where Jill attended Johns Hopkins'
School of Hygiene and Public Health, raised new possibilities. We trashed
the family finances, but it was a year of many gifts. The kids were happy
to spend uninterrupted time with their grandparents. They tried out new
schools and the boys followed the Ravens to a Super Bowl victory with their
favorite uncle. I wondered if the time had come to chuck medicine entirely.
But we came back after all. We had a house in Cincinnati and too many ties.
All the way home, I worried about re-entry, how I would handle being a
doctor again after so long a break.

As it happens, Khalil is the first patient on my schedule my first day back. The schedulers at the front desk knew what they were doing, making sure I started with him. I enter the room doubting my career in medicine. I don't know it yet, but I'll leave confident I can still do the job, perhaps enjoy it. Khalil transforms me, just like that. "Doctor Volck," he says, looking up from whatever else has caught his bubbling attention, that fabulous grin spreading across his thin, eager face. He says my name with inflections I can't hope to render, like Ella Fitzgerald scooping over and under the note, filling plain words with new, delicious meaning. But he's not sure of me yet, wondering, possibly, if I'm only back for a visit. He says nothing more until I ask. Then the dam breaks, and he floods me with a hundred important details.

"Doctor Volck, you were gone a long time. Where were you? Did you have fun? My dad says, 'hi.' Do you have new stickers? Are you going to listen to my heart?"

He has too many ideas to ask one at a time. A young Thelonious Monk at a piano of words, he piles one angular riff on the next, rarely finishing one before starting another, then circling back to jam on some unfinished invention. I sit down to listen, attentive, glowing. I look the same, I'm sure, when listening to Coltrane or Sarah Vaughan. Khalil speaks in music, and I listen.

But before Khalil does a thing, before he acknowledges my presence or speaks one heart-lifting note, Rhonda turns to me and says, "So you came back."

Yes.

* * * *

I once had lunch with Barry Moser, a gifted illustrator, artist, and lover of books, and we talked about hurtful words. He took a coffee cup in his hand and said, in his expansive drawl, "If all your childhood you're told this is a basket, it will always be that first in your mind. No matter how much you learn later, no matter how much you understand intellectually this is a coffee cup and not a basket, you'll still look at this and the first word that comes to your mind will be 'basket.' Our words form early. What comes after builds on that foundation."

If words alone determine behavior, racism is simply remedied: eliminate the words, and racism dies a well-deserved death. But words give form to feeling and momentum to intent without determining them. Not fully, at least. Change vocabulary, and so much remains: distrust, envy, fear. The roots of racism run deep, penetrating heart and mind. I change some of my actions, though not always my thoughts. I speak with care, but my heart still

festers. Warped desires and thoughts stand in full battle gear, weapons at the
ready for combat I never sought. They linger in the flesh, scars of deep and
wordless wounds I'm ashamed of and want to hide.

* * * *

"We don't use that word, *adopted*," Rhonda tells me. "*Adopted* is a Euro-
centric word. It puts him outside the family, the community. But he isn't
outside. He's in it." I sense what she's trying to tell me. I've written elsewhere
against the modern illusion that "biological children" are somehow more
legitimate, more "ours" than children welcomed some other way. Rhonda's
right: communal responsibility isn't an Anglo-American strong suit, a deficiency my language repeatedly betrays. In the words I'm given, however, I
confess *adoption* makes my heart sing. There's something about any adult in
this country and time, learning the hard, countercultural, and thoroughly
unprofitable practice of hospitality that sustains my tattered hope. I work
with several adoptive families, some of whom chose me for their pediatrician because I, too, am an adoptive parent. I don't know how supportive I
am. I'm not the support group kind. Yet we have a way of understanding,
these families and I. I do what I can and they do much for me. One adopted
family can make an entire day of struggle turn out right.

Some of my adoptive parents—more than you might expect—are single
women. Most of the parents are white. Most of the children are not. My office
waiting room would give a Klansman apoplexy. Khalil is African-American,
dark as the desert sky at midnight. Rhonda is lighter-skinned, illuminating
the office in flowing Guinea brocade. In the American parlance, however,
they are black and I am white. And Khalil is my favorite patient. Ever.

* * * *

Some would have called my parents prejudiced. That was the word then,
before most of us learned the word *racist*. *Prejudice* was used, as *racism* is
now, to describe what other people do. To call someone a racist distances
us from them. One's parents can be racist. We, however, pride ourselves
on overcoming all that. Some admit to lingering complicity, but to varying
effect. When Barry Moser says, "I'm a recovering racist," I hear the ongoing
struggle in his voice. When others say the same thing, I wonder if they're
scoring points among the enlightened who talk about such things.

How could my parents be anything but prejudiced? They were white
middle-class Americans. They bought a suburban house in the late 1940s in

what since has become a racially diverse neighborhood. Then it was white as the Ivory Soap my father's company advertised. When I, child of the late baby boom, said "black," they still said "negro." My parents never permitted disparaging slang or words of hate. Most of the racist language I heard in childhood came from television. I learned that vocabulary from Archie Bunker, even though the producers of the 1970s television show, *All in the Family*, were, I take it, spreading a thin, comforting veneer of white liberal tolerance over their audience. On television—then as now—appearance is everything. Archie's words, of course, were tame. Our next-door neighbors said the "n" word, but we understood them to be coarse and their father drank too much. Even so, I played with their youngest son until we grew too different to find anything to talk about.

Even the mild words, when I used them in public, earned disapproving scowls from my parents' friends. I once overheard my mother, in a conversation she understood to be private, tell how much she struggled against her prejudice. I shouldn't have listened in, but her words come back to me now as a gift, a tiny window into her own struggle, a mystery I wouldn't otherwise know. I sensed from her quavering tone how deeply she felt the shame of her thoughts. She never told me as much, but my television words, she said at another time, were no way to talk about anyone. Yet there was an unsettling abstraction to what adults said about race when I was a child. "Negroes," I heard my parents' friends say, "are welcome in the neighborhood as long as they keep up with the yard work." What lawn care skills the descendants of slaves might lack, they never explained. It seemed bad manners to ask.

There was a Chinese family at my school—the father was an optometrist—but no blacks. I had no idea what language was acceptable outside the relatively closed circle of my parents. Unspoken words were a transgression eating at me from the inside. One summer, I went on a Boy Scout trip to Washington, D. C. My troop and another from down the street went together. There were two black kids in the other troop. I forget their names, but the boy with glasses was quieter and smarter, and full of ideas for things to do. When the three of us were together, he was the natural, unchallenged leader. I liked being with them, and if it weren't for the words struggling to get out of my mouth, their skin would have been as irrelevant to me as last year's news.

For some reason, we spent part of our trip on a US Army base, staying in empty barracks. One afternoon—on what must have been a down day of the trip—we were just hanging out. I suggested we needed a name for our trio and offered up something like "Super Spade and the Gang." It was a word I'd never used before, never heard from a real person. It was a television word, a gift from Archie Bunker. The kid with glasses suddenly stopped playing, turned away from me, and paced. I knew straight away I'd done badly. For a moment, I hoped he hadn't really heard what I'd said. I wanted to take it all back, make what had just happened go differently. He looked really upset.

"I'm sorry," I said. "Maybe you can call me 'honkie.'" It was the worst word for a white person I knew.

"No," he said, his face crumpled, his voice with a new and bitter edge. That wouldn't work as a peace offering. Somehow—I don't remember how—we got to playing again, though it was never the same. I had ruined things with a word, and I couldn't even remember why I'd said it, except just to say it. Like Augustine, in *Confessions,* after he stole pears from his neighbor, I found no real joy in it, just willfulness.

Nearly four decades later, I feel that afternoon—the stacked, empty bunks of the Army barracks, afternoon light slanting through the windows, the look of anger and hurt on his face—rolling loosely in a pocket of my memory. I take it out from time to time, a jewel of guilt refracting the sunlight. I carry others in that same pocket, like the time I was playing upstairs and tipped over a large antique mirror. The sudden crash against the floor startled me in to silence, but my mother came up stairs to see if I was okay, which I was, at least physically. I shuddered, though, as she lifted the mirror, now face down on the floor, the intact wooden back offering some faint hope the glass itself remained unbroken. But it wasn't so. The floor was richly veined with shining, useless slivers and fragments lined with fine cracks like veins in an enormous leaf. My mother set the frame upright, sat down, and buried her head in hands. I don't know how long she wept, not saying a word. It seemed forever. She didn't hit or scold or punish me. She simply wept. I can still see, still hear her crying, decades later. She may have forgotten the whole thing years before her death. Surely she didn't want me to carry the guilt of that moment all these years, but I do.

And I still carry this whiteness. It's me. It's part of me. It's more than my skin.

* * * *

Khalil is in the hospital, four years after my return to Cincinnati. He has an unusual infection this time: odd bug, odd location. His fevers come and go with few other symptoms. My colleagues and I first attributed these to a virus, the pediatrician's backup explanation for most mysteries. When the fevers persisted, we rounded up the usual suspects: blood tests and cultures. His urine culture came back with a strange result, bacteria we took for a contaminant, something from his skin he hadn't fully washed away before giving us a sample. To make sure, we repeated the culture. The bacteria were still there. Rhonda is used to my befuddlement. Khalil confuses her, so why shouldn't he confuse me, too? She's not fond of the hospital, but resigns herself to it when Khalil must go. While treating Khalil's infection we've discovered a new problem, the latest in a list of anatomic anomalies that make my favorite patient so interesting. He has an unusually formed urinary tract, and this will require surgical correction. Rhonda knows there are more hospital stays in Khalil's future.

I visit Khalil whenever I can, even on days I'm not rounding for our group. He's clearly feeling better today, but he's still not ready to go home. I enter the room to find him sitting in bed watching television, his mother by the bedside. Televisions are always on in hospitals, but I find them distracting. I skew strongly towards visual learning: I'm a reader, a watcher. I'm not so good at listening. When the team presents at a patient's beside, I should devote my full attention to the medical student reading her history and physical. Why, then, do my eyes keep drifting toward Sponge Bob's adventures on the screen? I don't even like Sponge Bob. But the moving image grabs me. When I plan ahead, I turn the volume down and face away from the screen while the team is rounding.

I'm visiting Khalil, however, without the team. He's now enthralled by the onscreen gyrations of the Wiggles. I don't understand this show at all: four lanky white guys in turtlenecks prancing and singing with their pirate friend, Captain Feathersword? I try to distract Khalil, but he's rapt. I ask him about the show, but something in my tone must suggest disapproval.

"They're the Wiggles," he says, his voice raised. "Don't make fun."

I fumble through an exam, talk with Rhonda about the surgeon's plans and when they might be going home. Khalil pays me no mind.

I wash my hands, make ready to go, but can't resist another ploy for Khalil's attention.

"Some day, Khalil, you'll need to explain these guys to me. After all, don't they seem a little—well—white?"

Rhonda shoots me a quick smile. Khalil only glares.

* * * *

I want to know things: facts, explanations, origins. Information compensates for my social ineptitude. A downside of having what my wife calls a pathologically exact memory is that I can, off the top of my head, list for you a dozen of my most embarrassing social gaffes, stretching back four decades. It's evidence for what I already know: I'm a social dunce.

A man I know from the neighborhood brought his son, a senior in high school, to the office see me. The boy's just great: a good student, muscular, kind, looking forward to college. Both he and his dad are worried, though, about what they describe as social anxiety. "I can't think of things to say when I'm out with friends," he tells me. "I'm always trying to find words. I get so nervous because I don't know what to do. Sometimes it's just easier being alone." Because I'm his physician, we talked about ways to improve his social interactions. What I wanted to say to him, however, is, "Welcome to my life."

It's reassuring to hear how many writers say the same. Does standing forever outside the action in a social world make a writer or is it merely support the craft? Some people who feel like my patient generously lubricate themselves with alcohol at or even before social encounters. Many writers turn to alcohol during their careers, too, but I've never heard of one who thought much of the stuff he wrote while drunk. Honest writing, like honest love, is too demanding, calling us, at the same time, into and out of the self. Alcohol never gets us past appearances.

Routines help. Familiar situations help a lot. Once I get the patter down, I know how to do the small talk. It helps that I acted onstage in school and inherited my father's bass voice, affording the illusion of confidence. But I'm forever looking for the intellectual key, the knowing technique that makes for confidence, rather than merely its appearance.

I once said all this to a woman I know, a brilliant and sensitive physician whose opinion I trust. What I said was, "I always imagine everyone else knows how to behave and I don't. It's like I missed the meeting when the rules of etiquette were passed out. I'm always guessing at what to do, what to say, and I end up thinking I offended someone who's too polite to tell me, even if everyone else already knows."

The woman whose opinion I trusted looked at me hard and said, "You can't feel that way. Only women feel that way."

* * * *

"Yes, you told me you write," Rhonda says. She and I are talking about what I do on days I'm not in the office, seeing patients. I make a point of saying that inpatient rounds and family responsibilities often cut deeply into my writing time. I didn't want her to think I'm a slacker. I want to tell her that writing keeps the scattering threads of my life in some order, but I think she already knows.

The next time she brings Khalil to the office, she has a copy of her play. It's about four African-American women getting together and talking. I admire her skill at dialogue, each spoken line a discovery, another step forward. Rhonda knows how to listen, knows what to listen for. If only I had her ear.

Reading her play is like sitting in a busy restaurant and overhearing a great conversation at the next table. Why couldn't I be that witty? I sometimes ask myself if white people are simply boring, or if they just seem that way to me after spending so much of my life among them. I suppose the familiar eventually grows stale, especially for those trained by television to never be satisfied with what we have.

This day Rhonda gives me her script, I have twenty patients scheduled for office visits. Their ages skew towards infancy, though a number of school kids are in the bunch. Most are African-American, and most of the talking, especially when I'm seeing the very young ones, will be between me and the patient's mother. We have four registered nurses and two nursing aides in the office. Half of them are African-American. They're the ones I talk with when things are slow. I spend most of my working day in the company of black women.

Put that way, it sounds like another showy display of liberal piety, the way some talk of their new, rechargeable electric sedan as if planetary survival has been secured by this one, shrewd purchase. Yes, I spend my days with African-American women, but I do so because of my privileged place as a doctor. It's a security that cuts both ways: granting me astonishing access to personal details and a familiarity with people I'd otherwise never stop to talk with, while leaving me forever outside of those lives, separated as often by class or education as by skin color.

When I lived on the Navajo Reservation, I knew no matter how long I stayed, I would always be a visitor from somewhere else. I also saw up close how sad and parasitic wannabes are, how protestations of oceanic tolerance never change who you are and where you come from. When I'm asked what I learned from my years on the Reservation, I usually say, "That I'm not Indian; not even in a past life."

That last bit usually elicits a double take, but it's not a throw away line. I've met people insistent on exotic past selves—usually noble, often famous—in their earlier incarnations. I've yet to meet someone who was a starving serf in a forgotten fiefdom. Dead Indians, it turns out, are hot commodities among those seeking gratifying tales of preexistence. Not content with stealing native land, language, and culture, the wannabes—who are

mostly white, materially comfortable, and well educated—now steal ancestors. There's something quintessentially American about descendants of
European immigrants claiming they've outgrown their own religious and
cultural heritage while spiritually raping another and wielding the trendy
vocabulary of consumerist pseudo-Buddhism as their weapon of choice. I
can't imagine how conscientious Buddhists feel about the misuse of their
tradition by ill-informed North Americans. I know it doesn't go over well
with Indians.

* * * *

Before we welcomed Maria into our family, before Jill and I travelled to
Guatemala to bring her home, before her presence made us a transracial
family, I had the unnoticed and unsought-after privilege of deciding, on any
given day, whether or not to be conscious of racism. Before Maria, I could,
if I chose, denounce gross forms of bigotry, march in the right parades, and
display my bourgeois liberal credentials for all to admire. Or not. I could, in
fact, simply mind what I was taught to call "my own business." My periodic
failure to notice racism, much less respond to it, did me no visible harm. But
when Jill and I stepped into the concourse of what was then the Houston
Intercontinental Airport, carrying our daughter as the newest immigrant
to the United States, I saw that people who looked like Jill and me walked
briskly to their flights while those who looked like Maria pushed brooms.
It was like having distorting eyeglasses, of which I'd until then been un-
aware, suddenly fall from my face and shatter on the concourse floor. I saw
more clearly, but with an acute sense of loss, a new vulnerability. Racism,
wherever I now encounter it—even in myself—wounds my daughter, and
through her, wounds me.

I love my daughter as a father cannot help but love—with all my
heart—but how do I honor her when I know fragments of my heart are,
by virtue of my upbringing, irreformably racist. "Who," as Aleksandr Solzhenitsyn writes in *The Gulag Archipelago*, "is willing to destroy a piece of
his own heart?"[1]

* * * *

I'm not black. I'm not Latina. I'm not poor, illiterate, Navajo, or Hopi. I'm
a white doctor, sitting in an examining room with Khalil and Rhonda, and
we're just talking. For now, I don't feel like an outsider. I haven't missed the

---

1. Solzhenitsyn, *The Gulag Archipelago*, volume 1, 168.

meeting where the rules were handed out. Khalil's in his school uniform, telling me about his teacher, about how he wears his ostomy bag so it doesn't irritate his skin, about plans for his birthday. I'll tell him about my kids, about my son who's come with me to visit Khalil in the hospital and who asks about him from time to time, about the stories my other son tells, about my daughter's fascination with rocks and fossils.

Race is still here, stealing oxygen from the room. So, too, are the wounds and words. Memories cut me with glinting, mirrored edges I can't help but touch. There's too much going on in my head. I mentally juggle baskets and cups, flailing to keep them separate. I'm hoping the ugly stains on my heart aren't as obvious to Khali, Rhonda, and Maria as they are to me. But I'm also here—present in body—just sitting and talking with my favorite patient.

My job wears me down, but moments like these keep me from leaving. I almost left that year in Baltimore, but I came back. I came back for all sorts of reasons: family, because I had bills to pay, because I didn't have anything else worked out yet. I came back, and I'm where I need to be. I'm sitting in a room, talking to Khalil and Rhonda and, just for now, there's no other place I'd rather be.

Chapter Eleven

Embodying the Word

*Cincinnati, Ohio/Departamento
de Yoro, Honduras*

FOR OVER A DECADE, I co-taught an annual medical student elective in literature and medicine. We started each class with a writing exercise, a prompt—usually from the text we're about to discuss—to which the students responded, telling stories from their clinical experience. They had fifteen or twenty minutes to write. Some touched pen to paper immediately, pouring memories on the page. Others stared blankly or with a pinched look of concern until words came at last. Then each student read his or her vignette aloud. As a group, we paused to respond whenever a familiar scene, nagging question, or evocative phrase struck home. It was different every time: a troubling experience with an insensitive doctor, a private struggle to overcome some misunderstanding, or the kindness of a patient in adversity. Only after everyone spoke did we turn to the book at hand. Our goal was to connect what we read to our lives as physicians.

We encouraged reading as engagement, asking more of a book than mere diversion to pass the time; more than edification, to leave us "better-read"; and more than a mass of data awaiting interpretation. I wanted them to like what we read, but didn't insist on it. I'd much rather students wrestle with a book than say nice things they don't mean. Disliking an author—and saying why—beats empty pleasantries any day.

Like the practice of diagnosis through history-taking and physical exam, engaging what we read demands patience, attention, and discipline. Some books, of course, prove better reading than others. Telling the keepers from the ones best thrown back—that's the trick. I spoke about this with a friend and mentor who divides her time between writing, family, and commercial fishing. As we brushed away the early morning chill outside a cabin on Puget Sound, the conversation turned to her own education in writing. She described authors who mistook ugliness for profundity, and intricate prose that, for all its style and flash, was stillborn.

I was newer to the craft and unsure what to say, so I mumbled something about narcissism in contemporary poetry, how I no longer understand what passes for good or bad. "I have favorites," I conceded, "the few I return to again and again, but there's so much I don't connect with. As arrogant as it sounds, I don't have time for words that stay on the page."

I startled at what I'd just said. Hopelessly self-referential, I appeared to demand more from a book than its reader, but that gets things backwards. For words to leave the page, they need somewhere to go. That demands at least as much of the reader as the text. I can, for instance, search Smith's *Recognizable Patterns of Human Malformation*, a standard text on congenital disorders, find the entry on a condition called "Williams Syndrome," and read about the characteristic "elfin" face (full cheeks, wide mouth, broad, upturned nose), the associated intellectual deficits, increased blood calcium levels in infancy, a rare heart defect called supravalvular aortic stenosis, and the development in the teenage years of a talkative manner (the so-called "cocktail party personality"). It's interesting, but remains words on a page without someone to embody them.

The practical goal of medical reading is to link the words we read to the bodies we care for. When I think of Williams Syndrome, what I see isn't a page in a book, but the baby I helped diagnose while I was still a pediatric intern. He'd been admitted to the hospital for poor weight gain, and his initial laboratory work showed abnormally high blood calcium. The senior resident chuckled when I first mentioned the possibility of Williams Syndrome. She'd seen book-smart interns shinny out on slender diagnostic limbs before, and reminded me that the unfortunate thing about uncommon diagnoses is how uncommon they are. Her skepticism spurred in me an eagerness to prove my hunch right. I didn't know it then, but it would be the lone diagnostic coup of my entire residency.

The memories of how I built my case and won others over are now shadowy and fragmented: a genetics consult, a conversation with a cardiologist, more testing. What I remember clearly, though, is a conference held for the family, explaining to them the diagnosis and its long-term implications.

The baby's father was a construction worker from the west side of Cleveland who moved his family from West Virginia in search of a better life. He was still young, with wiry, muscular forearms, but his face was deeply lined, like the cracked clay bed of a drained pond. In well-worn jeans and a flannel shirt, he sat in deferential silence at the table while platoons of white-coated doctors, genetic counselors, and social workers shared their knowledge and recommendations. The experts chose their words carefully, hoping to inform without confusion or offense. When talk turned to the possibility of developmental delay—what at the time was called mental retardation—the father's expression grew at once softer and more serious.

"Are you telling me my boy's gonna be a slow learner?" he asked.

There followed a brief, awkward silence. No one enjoys telling parents about a child's likely mental insufficiency.

"Yes," the geneticist said, "You could put it that way."

"Well, that's okay," he said with a slight nod," I'm a slow learner, too."

Tension leaked from the room like air from a balloon. A father with little formal education but more life experience than we could guess had just gone out of his way to put a roomful of credentialed professionals at ease. Since then, when I read about Williams Syndrome, the words refuse to stay on the page. They live in body of a young boy and in the kindness of his father: small treasures I put together with what the words say.

Some patients appear to have "read the textbook"—displaying classic signs and symptoms—like Paul, the child I diagnosed with diabetes when Joy, his mother, brought him on his first visit to my office. First appointments are generally spent gathering information, reviewing the medical history and exam, and discussing practices to maintain good health. Joy, however, had more urgent concerns. She told me of her son's worsening problems, beginning with what had seemed a mild viral illness. Since then, Paul had steadily lost weight. He was often tired and always thirsty. He ran to the bathroom frequently—even wetting the bed at night, a problem he hadn't had for years. I asked a few more questions and performed a cursory exam before directing Paul don the hallway to provide a urine sample and to have his blood sugar tested. His urine was positive for glucose and ketones. His blood sugar was nearly 300.

Osler and Laennec said, "Listen to the patient. He is giving you the diagnosis." Paul's body shouted his condition: New Onset Type One Diabetes. No doctor likes to make an unwelcome, life-changing diagnosis. I certainly didn't, especially with a family I'd just met. But Paul embodied nearly every word I remembered reading about the clinical diagnosis of diabetes. In both cases—Paul's and the boy with Williams Syndrome—the challenge was in the leap from page to person. Even in the best of situations, that leap requires a certain amount of faith in one's capacity to interpret and apply a text.

I've had skilled mentors in medicine. Some were the best in their fields. Many were kind and generous. The textbooks and journal articles they recommended contained essential information—an ignorant physician is a danger to his patients—and I studied them with relish. But I learn at least as much from patient encounters and the stories told in exam rooms. Better doctors than I have said as much. Better writers, too.

Almost all the books that schooled me in the fraught world of doctor-patient encounters came from outside the peer-reviewed medical canon: short stories by William Carlos Williams, novels by Shusaku Endo and Albert Camus, memoirs by Abraham Verghese, nonfiction by Anne Fadiman—narratives of all sorts. To learn about kindness in difficult circumstances, there was Dorothea Brooke in *Middlemarch* or Stephen Kumalo in *Cry, The Beloved Country*. Reminders of how professionalism without affection—or common sense—corrupts judgment came from the Chancery functionaries in *Bleak House* or Stevens, the butler, in *The Remains of the Day*. To discover harsh realities my patients knew better than I, there was Ralph Ellison's nameless *Invisible Man* or Tayo, the haunted Laguna veteran in *Ceremony*. Mostly, though, I read what interested me. If I found myself still turning a scene from book in my mind two weeks after having finished reading, the words had left their mark.

With time, though, I wondered if some ways of reading might prove better at lifting words from the page. When I learned to perform a physical exam, I'd never seriously considered *not* submitting to the example of my masters. I followed their lead or failed the course. I used my hands, ears, and eyes according to their example. I don't do a complete physical exam on every patient I see. A follow-up visit for school-related problems may not require one. Yet I've done thorough exams often enough to know their value, and I measure their utility and appropriateness based on the situation at hand. Was I willing to do likewise when it came to reading words instead of bodies? What I lacked was a practice on which to build my reading, a place to start from.

I don't recall when I first learned of *lectio divina*, a reading practice rooted in Christian monasticism still followed by contemporary Benedictine monks, nuns, and laypersons. A centuries-old contemplative practice seems an unlikely model for a doctor in a teaching hospital, but when I seek words that jump from the page, *lectio* helps.

Lectio divina, like the examination of the abdomen, is traditionally divided into four parts: *lectio* (reading), *meditatio* (meditation), *oratio*
(prayer), and *contemplatio* (contemplation). *Lectio divina* hasn't changed
much over the centuries. Some traditions are hard to improve upon. Simply
put, it asks the reader to attend, to notice the details of the text and name
the responses they engender. In *lectio,* a passage is read slowly, paused over,
and read again—aloud, if possible, engaging the body through eye, mouth,
and ear. What words, phrases, or images stand out? Given time, attention
drifts from holy-sounding words toward the mundane and familiar, made
suddenly strange: "mud," "five smooth stones," "afraid," "loaves and fishes."
The mystics insist it's in earthy realities that the Maker of the Universe hides.

In *meditatio,* the passage is considered in relation to the reader's life.
How does today's reading apply? Don't mar the text with theoretical abstraction or aggressive interpretation. This is a conversation to be entered,
not a puzzle in need of a solution. *Oratio* is where true conversation begins,
an opening of the heart in prayer. What needs to be said? What response is
called for? Keep the intellect on a short leash. Go with the gut. *Contemplatio*
is the attentive silence that follows, when the fleshy confluence of mind and
heart—what Orthodox mystics call *nous*– stands before Divine mystery:
receptive, aware, listening. A quick summary of the steps goes, "Reading
seeks, meditation finds, prayer asks, and contemplation feels." In *lectio
divina,* feeling isn't the intellect's enemy, but its fulfillment.

The Rule of Saint Benedict (the founding document of Western monasticism), in use since the sixth century, opens with the phrase, "*Obsculta,
o fili, præcepta magistri, et inclina aurem cordis tui.*" "Listen, O son, to the
Master's teaching, and bend the ear of your heart." Related to the word with
which Benedict begins his Rule is the Latin compound verb *ob-audire,* an
attentive and embodied form of listening, from which English derives the
word *obedience.* That's an unappealing word for modern readers. I'm not
suggesting that all texts should be received unquestioningly. Benedict's en-
dorsement of "prayerful reading" concerned texts recognized as authoritative, or at least beneficial, for the community. Someone like me, with tastes
and choices astronomically larger than the library of a medieval monastery,
will likely read *Anna Karenina* differently than a Tony Hillerman mystery,
though I can enjoy, attend to, and learn from both. Similarly, the reader
brings herself, including all she's read, experienced, suffered from, and wondered about, to what she reads.

It sounds deceptively cerebral, but listening and reading are embodied actions: words received through physical senses, bending the ear of
the heart. A friend of mine teaches at a seminary in California and leads
classes and workshops in *lectio divina.* A day or so into the course, he

asks learners if they've noticed any changes in their social dynamics. The most common responses include, "We're listening better and talking less," or "We're more present to one another than when we started." Practices become habits. What my own attempts at *lectio divina* offer is a habit of presence and focused attention. *Lectio* acknowledges some written words are important enough to demand this. My patients' spoken words deserve the same. Both "presence," from the Latin root "to be before or at hand," and attention, "to stretch toward," engage the body. There are, I know, centuries-old caricatures reducing monasticism to a set of crude dualisms, punishing the body in favor of the spiritual or despising the entire world in pursuit of individual sanctity. The Rule of St. Benedict, however, is deeply concerned with communal habits of the body: eating together and sleeping alone, praying, reading, singing, and working. Special attention is given to hospitality: meeting the material needs of strangers and guests. When the monk sits or stands at *lectio divina*, he doesn't reject the body. He labors to remain present to the word.

Some might call *lectio divina* "mindful reading," using vocabulary associated with Eastern traditions. Insofar as "mindful" means focused attention on present reality—now, here, this—it's a helpful term. In my experience, though, North Americans already overvalue the mind, and particularly the will. We attend to things instrumentally, to achieve an intended purpose. We make the body serve the mind. Yet Eastern practices commonly associated with "mindfulness" necessarily involve the body: sitting, chanting, breathing, fasting, and living simply. The chief enemy of contemplation is distraction, "letting the mind wander." The difficulty I have with attention lies in remaining where the body is now, rather than wandering somewhere else and in some other time. I'm grateful to the Orthodox mystics who enlarged the Greek word, *nous*—often translated simply as "mind"—to embody what Orthodox poet Scott Cairns calls "the heart's intellective aptitude" at "that queer, cool confluence of breath/and blood."[1]

I've met grumpy monks, but they're exceptions. Most are visibly content. The best are joyful, unafraid, and fully present, conversing with me as if I were the most important person in the world. Wise monks seek a necessary balance: guarding their solitude while drawing on lifelong habits of hospitality to receive guests and words kindly, attentively, convivially. Among the fruits of hospitality is getting to know one's guests, pushing past first impressions to deeper understanding. Similarly, *lectio divina* encourages the

---

1. Cairns, "Adventures in New Testament Greek: *Nous*" in *Slow Pilgrim: The Collected Poems*, 183.

reader or hearer to push past surface readings through the interplay of text and attentive recipient.

Lectio divina doesn't end in listening or reading. *Laborare et orare* is the Benedictine motto: "work and prayer." With practice, the seams between reading and response fade into the fabric of a life. Word becomes flesh in the daily performance of Scripture. In my attempts to engage text and tradition, I've learned that performing the word isn't something only monks and nuns do. In my reading of words that matter, as in my reading of the body in physical exam, I must respond.

For much of human history, houses of prayer and houses of healing were closely connected. Hospitals began as *xenones* in the Christian East and hospices in the medieval West: houses of hospitality for the sick, the poor, and the pilgrim. In recent centuries, however, things have changed. No one I know checks into the hospital for quiet contemplation. If I arrive in the Emergency Department complaining of crushing chest pain that started in my left shoulder, I want the medical team to treat my heart attack right away, not stand idly by pondering what phrases in my chief complaint resonate with their life. There are occasions in medicine where rapid and efficient response is needed to save a life. That's why doctors and nurses frequently practice advanced life support techniques. We must respond quickly if delay means death.

Yet most medical practice requires a more deliberate pace. Doctors listen to the patient and read the chart to reach a diagnosis and propose a treatment plan. Medical training emphasizes utilitarian aspects of the patient's story: the history upon which doctors impose useable significance. The skills are necessary, if often insufficient. A doctor in training, anxious to prove herself, can't help but view the patient's story as basic raw material in need of a prepared mind to solve the diagnostic puzzle. She will come, with experience and time, to understand that humans are rarely simple and few tell their stories straightforwardly.

Doctors enter the patient's room with a goal in mind. The family waits there with a sick child. Medicine is an applied science, wedding technology and knowledge to make things happen—or keep them from happening. We listen to histories not much differently than we read textbooks or consult online evidence-based resources for the latest information on best practices. We seek reliable, efficient means toward desired outcomes. Physicians make things happen in the physical world in service to the bodies of patients. The realities of modern medical care, however, make that difficult.

At Cincinnati Children's, we use "family-centered rounds" when seeing inpatients. The medical team—ideally the entire range of interested decision-makers: nurses, interns, residents, attendings, therapists, consultants, and parents—gathers at the patient's bedside to review the hospital course and plan the day ahead. The presenting intern speaks directly to the parent in everyday language, explaining technical terms as they arise and inviting the parent to correct any part of the history we've gotten wrong. The goal is to arrive at a common understanding and an agreed-upon plan. The family-centered aspect is a challenge for anyone captivated by the efficient vocabulary of the medical profession or unused to including parents in the messy process of assessing relevant medical information. That's why we practice.

But the ideal is hard to sustain. It's 8:15 am and the team crowds into a darkened patient room on A6 South, a general pediatrics inpatient unit. There are nine of us: a senior resident, three interns, three medical students, the patient's nurse, and me, the attending physician. We've wheeled three laptop computers on mobile stands into the room as well. Tori, the fifteen month-old we've come to see, awakens as we enter and starts to cry, pulling at the oxygen cannula at her nose and reaching through the bars of her crib for her parents. Tori's mother rises from the bedside couch to comfort her while Dad rubs his sleepy eyes. The presenting intern starts to tell Tori's story. She's doing a good job, speaking to the parents without lapsing into Medspeak, but it's not clear if they're awake enough to understand. Tori arrived after midnight and the parents' first chance to sleep was four a.m. No one slept well. The senior resident eyes Tori's breathing as he listens for the intern's assessment and plan, which he will comment on. Another intern types new orders into a computer while a third updates the patient's hospital summary for discharge. The medical students hear that Tori has an interesting heart murmur. One student asks Tori's parents if she can listen to her chest, too. They stare at first, then nod approval. The students line up at bedside. Pagers go off. Monitor alarms sound. The nurse is called away to care for another patient. I stay in the corner by the door, letting the team show me what they can do. I know if I stand up front the parents and intern will defer to me, not allowing the senor resident to make his own decisions before I chime in. In front is also directly in line with the television screen, where my all-too-visual attention will turn to Dora the Explorer as a moth is drawn to flame. In my corner, I close my eyes, focus on the ongoing conversation, and try not to think about the fifteen other inpatients we still must see before noon.

Beneath these tasks and distractions lurk the dynamics of Tori's illness. Her mother is worried. This is her third hospitalization in two months, each for a respiratory infection severe enough to require supplemental oxygen. Mom wants to know why Tori keeps getting sick. She fears we're missing something when the intern explains it's another viral infection. She wants

Tori to get and stay better, and grasps for explanations to restore a sense of control. She's learning the First Law of Parenthood: she's not in control. We all want Tori to get better, for her family to go home and get on with their lives, but she isn't ready. The family's anxiety over what we might be missing and their fear for Tori's future widen the existing power gap between them and us—the medical professionals who speak in mystifying jargon, wield near-magical technology, and spend long hours far from the patient's room. Emotions gather like storm clouds, garbling communication and turning small misunderstandings into full-scale battles.

The intern worries about making the right diagnosis, proposing an appropriate plan, making that plan happen, getting Tori out of the hospital, and impressing me enough to earn a good evaluation. She knows surprising new information may arise at any time, plans may change, and attending physicians are often gruff. She hopes her interactions with Tori's parents remain—if not pleasant—then at least clear and efficient, with their words and concerns easily translated into medical language. But if Tori's parents don't follow the expected pattern or the clouds of stress and mistrust finally burst, the intern will want nothing so urgently as to get out of the room.

It's precisely then that presence is needed: a practice to banish distraction, dial down emotion, return attention to the exchange happening right now, and note my responses—mental and physical. I like nearly all my patients, so when I'm in a room with a family and the hair on the back of my neck rises like the hackles on a German Shepherd or my eyes search for the doorknob, something odd is happening. Often it's another instance of what philosopher of science Michael Polanyi called "tacit knowledge": the awareness of something quite real, though resistant to articulation. Analysis will help in the long run, but what's required right now is full attention. That's when I live into the role of *attending* physician. If I'm in the hospital, watching the team present, I stop slouching in the corner and step forward. If I'm seeing my patient in an examining room, I straighten my spine and face the family as directly as possible. My body grows fully engaged, my senses focus on the words, gestures, and posture of those speaking. I choose words carefully, strain to listen, and clarify ambiguities before offering my opinion. It's an encounter I'll mull over long afterward.

I try to model this for learners. I remind them later that listening to the patient includes noting silences between words and asking awkward questions. Difficult encounters become opportunities for understanding if one knows how to respond. Without practices of attentive presence, the patient's real concerns will be overlooked, important information remain hidden, diagnoses missed, and complex therapies wasted.

I also teach residents in an elective we call "Poverty, Justice, and Health." We introduce learners to what's called "poverty medicine": the challenges and strengths of people in economic poverty whose medical problems are as much the product of large social factors as they are of individual choices or microscopic pathogens. Our residents see patients in inner-city clinics, visit homeless shelters and emergency food banks, accompany a family applying for Medicaid, and learn from social workers, public health professionals, and church volunteers what it's like to patch the walking wounded and send them back on the street. For many, it's eye opening, their first encounter outside the Emergency Department with patients whose resources and options are pitifully few. They begin to grasp why certain patients can't do what's medically necessary to get better. They discover things technology and good intentions can't fix.

On Friday mornings, our learners gather with a faculty mentor and share stories from the week. These aren't tales of medical successes or therapeutic breakthroughs, but stories about presence during patient encounters, of listening for the story hidden in the medical complaint.

"At the downtown clinic," one resident said, "I saw a three-month-old in for her first visit. She hadn't seen a doctor since birth. The mom looked real young—I forget how old she was—and she had four other kids at home. She worked the third shift and looked absolutely exhausted. She was grateful for any help she got with the children, and most of that came from her mother.

"After examining the baby, I asked her, 'If there's one thing in the world we could do right now to help you with your baby, what would it be?'

"She said, 'I need diapers.'"

"I asked if there was anything else she needed—money, vouchers, a ride home—but all she wanted were diapers. She was incredibly grateful when we handed her a bagful. I'm trained in all this high-powered medical care, and all she really wanted from me were diapers."

Another resident shared her own feelings of anger:

"It was late on a busy afternoon in the clinic, and I entered the exam room to find a young mother busily texting away on her cell phone.

"It had been nine months since the mom brought her baby to the clinic, and the infant was behind on all her shots. The baby had an ear infection and was miserable, but the mom wouldn't calm her, help with the exam, or focus on what was happening. She said she needed to leave soon for another appointment."

That's when the resident decided to stop, take a breath, and ask the young woman how she was doing. She discovered the mother's husband was in jail, forcing her to quit her job to care for the kids. She hadn't brought the baby in because she'd lost her health insurance and her car, and the urgent appointment was to see her husband before visiting hours ended.

"Until then," said the resident, "I hadn't stopped to consider the story behind her attitude. That made all the difference in how I listened to her, what we talked about, and what I responded to as a doctor. And maybe it helped the mom, too, just saying aloud what she saw as the real problem."

In both stories, the turning point was an open-ended question and readiness to remain present, listening, to another person's revelation. The residents no longer simply heard what was said; they *felt* it, too.

The traditional medical history and physical begins with a chief complaint—what the patient perceives as the problem requiring attention—before addressing that complaint with medical knowledge and technology. Nowadays, patient histories often leave out the chief complaint, skipping over the patient's words and falling headlong into medical verbiage. "My stomach hurts" becomes, "This seven year old male presents with a two-day history of abdominal pain, vomiting, and nonbloody, nonbilious diarrhea." Perhaps the chief complaint remains in robust health elsewhere, but where I teach, it's vanishing like the tail on a tadpole.

What's lost is this: the chief complaint is an acknowledgment, however brief, that the first narrator of the patient's illness is the patient—or, in pediatrics, the parent. By asking the question, "What's wrong?" the physician enters the patient's suffering—a threshold many fear to cross. It's not a new fear and not limited to doctors. "What's wrong?" is the question Parzival, the Grail Knight of medieval legend, desperately needed to ask Anfortas, the mysteriously wounded Fisher King. Parzival was warned against excessive curiosity before he first met Anfortas, whose painful wound incapacitated him. As long as Parzival maintained a respectful reticence, the King lay unhealed and suffering. Parzival himself suffered mightily before another opportunity arose to ask the fateful question, an interval during which he learns the crucial difference between curiosity and compassion, the latter word coming from the Latin, "to suffer with." There are times when suffering-with is the most anyone can do.

In the mountain clinics of rural Honduras, where every medicine and piece of equipment arrives by pickup or is carried on our backs, there's no way to bring all we want or need. Before heading out, we listen to the locals, ask doctors who've been before, and assemble our materials accordingly. Tylenol and Motrin, vitamins and antibiotics, soaps and toothbrushes are stuffed into plastic bags and shoved into backpacks. We make room for a scale, thermometer, paper and pens, as well as personal medical equipment:

stethoscopes, flashlights, blood pressure cuffs. Whatever else comes along is the result of an educated guess.

In the field, we fit what we have to the needs at hand. There are always surprises, unexpected injuries, and conditions unaccounted for. If there's time and transportation, we refer these to base clinic. Otherwise, we improvise. A piece of wood paired with cloth and tape will splint a broken limb. A large bandana makes a sling. Pain relievers cover a multitude of sins.

Honduran *campesinos* know about improvisation and making do. If a woman in labor can't walk to the clinic, she's brought by "bamboolance": a hammock strung on a long bamboo pole, carried by men at each end. Elderly patients travel in the bed of a truck or on the back of a mule. Families use home remedies when the doctor's far away. What North Americans see as crippling conditions, rural Hondurans treat as mere inconvenience. Yet there are times when even Honduran ingenuity fails.

Above the village of Llano de Balas, a winding footpath leading seemingly nowhere unexpectedly spills onto an abandoned soccer field. The spectacular view is enjoyed chiefly by cattle grazing near crumbling goalposts, but a small hut stands past a stone wall on the far side. Its walls are sticks and mud, the thatched roof dark with smoke from many cooking fires and probably crawling with reduviid beetles, insect carriers for the microscopic parasite causing Chagas disease, a chronic infection that's potentially fatal if not treated in its early stages. We'd been asked by some villagers below to visit the elderly couple living there. Our medical team was small—a resident and a medical student, a nursing student, my son, Peter, now in high school, and me. We were lightly equipped, having left most of our supplies in the village schoolhouse. It was a cloudless afternoon, and we saw no one moving in or around the house until we were very close, when a woman came to the window and gestured us toward the side door. Outside stood a small wooden cross, inscribed with the name of her only son, who had died several years before. Chickens cackled in the shade. A small fire burned under a pot.

I never learned how long the woman who lived there had hearing problems, but she'd grown completely deaf. She read lips, though, and could follow along if we kept to Spanish. She laughed when she discovered the medical student was named Julie, close enough to her own name of Julia to insist on an embrace. Julia's husband had been blind from cataracts for two years. How the two of them communicated is a mystery, but they managed, our incomprehension notwithstanding.

He had worked fields his whole life and was proud of his abilities as a farmer, but disability and a growing need of assistance discouraged him. He sat on a low wooden bench rubbing his aching joints. A chicken pecked at the ground underneath, a string tied to one leg to keep the bird from stray-ing. The man blamed his blindness on blowing sand that irritated his eyes while farming, but he spoke without hint of self-pity. All he wanted was to farm again, and for that he needed to see.

We were reasonably confident about his diagnosis of cataracts. He'd been previously evaluated by a visiting doctor who recommended an oph-thalmologist in El Progreso, hundreds of miles away. He could get the nec-essary surgery there, but he must first arrange transportation and a place to stay in town before and after the procedures. He had no money and no relatives in El Progreso. Even if he did, how would he make the treacherous hike down the switchbacks to Llano de Balas, then up the mountain and over the ridge to the road, from which, at last, he could take a bus? It takes a fit, sighted person half a day to walk that route. For him, who knew? And what would his wife do in his absence? Neighbors could take her in or look after her, but he'd worry about her, so far away and without his help. And even if they could go together, carried by bamboolance or riding on mules, this house was the only place they had ever known. Central American cities are rarely hospitable to penniless strangers. How these two would survive without relations or friends was anyone's guess.

We listened intently and asked polite questions, but it was clear we weren't going to improvise a way out of this. We offered halfhearted sug-gestions, faces falling even as we spoke. Yet when I stepped away to mull things over, I saw what the others were doing. They stood erect, leaned in to better hear what was said. Those with better Spanish repeated the couple's words aloud, first in Spanish and then in English, making sure the rest un-derstood. Everyone spoke slowly, visibly considering what they were about to say. Even my teenage son carried himself with dignity, attending to what these two—one blind, one deaf; both scarred by hard living—had to share. The couple thanked us repeatedly for coming. We stayed awhile, enjoying each other's company. We took photos. Julia laughed aloud at her digital image. We had nothing to fix their problems but, as if to relieve our collec-tive conscience, left a bottle of Ibuprofen tablets and several bars of soap. Then we said our farewells and started back, descending the switchbacks in silence. No one spoke for a long time after.

From the point of view of scientific medicine—always on the search for pragmatic solutions—we'd done nothing for them. We discussed possi-ble treatment options, but these were words, not actions. Far from expensive technology, we exerted none of our vaunted control power, made no signifi-cant changes. And when, on our return to base clinic, we asked members of the committee for money to bring the couple to El Progreso, they told us of equally pressing needs, closer to home, for which they had neither funds nor material resources.

Under the circumstances, we had given them all we could: our time, our presence, our attention. We visited them in their home. We listened to their stories. We stood in witness. We carry them in memory. In a brief intersection of radically different lives, we acknowledged one another's frail humanity. That was our therapy, a word from the Greek, *therapon*, "one who attends." As medical professionals, we had come wanting to do so much more.

Chapter Twelve

Roberto and Jenrry

Departamento de Intibucá, Honduras

"WE'RE HERE?"

I startled from fitful dozing as the truck engine cut off. Miguel, the Honduran doctor who drove the eight hours from Tegucigalpa, smiled at my confusion. Over his shoulder, through the truck window, I saw the familiar rust and yellow tiles of the clinic steps. We were in the clinic compound at Santa Lucia. I'd been taken by surprise again.

Had I been paying attention, I would have recognized the tidy houses lining the road as we passed through Magdalena, a morning's walk to the north. That came after four hours of rocky, dirt highway—rarely wide enough for two trucks—meandering its dusty way from the pines of La Esperanza to the steamy Rio Torola and onward to El Salvador. As ridge after bluish mountain ridge faded in the haze, I sprawled in my seat half awake, unable to read or truly sleep, unsettled in the rising heat. I opened my eyes on occasion, noting the passing buildings and valleys, then slumbered again, thinking about the work accumulating in my absence, back in the States. Now I was at *Clinica Hombro a Hombro*. It was time to start the work I'd come all this way to do.

Regular clinic hours were over, but the gates stood open. Don Beto, policing the yard, flashed a toothy grin beneath his dark cowboy hat as Miguel stepped from the driver's seat. By the time I, too, set foot on the gravelly driveway, Don Beto was already pulling luggage from the flatbed.

We exchange relaxed Honduran "*buen' dias*" and started upstairs. Just past the wooden clinic doors stood Ed, looking as pleased to see me as I him.

"Brian! We've been waiting for a pediatrician to get here. There's a kid we want you to see."

"Serious?" I asked, not quite ready after the long ride to assume the role of consulting physician.

"He's got severe malnutrition. Been here a few days already. He's got us worried, but he's reasonably stable. Why don't you get settled now and you can see him a little later?"

Ed's graying beard, bright eyes, and ready smile afforded him a wise, experienced look. Ed and his wife, Candace, traveled from Pennsylvania to Central America for medical work over many years. Ed's stateside responsibilities as a family physician include migrant health and tuberculosis treatment. Candace trains midwives in the United States and Guatemala. Both speak fluent Spanish and practice the healing arts with passion and skill. Family practitioners sometimes get a bad rap from other specialists as superficially trained and insufficiently focused. If you really want to know what you're doing, they say, you must specialize, limit your scope. Ed destroyed that myth.

Once, when I worked with Ed in another Honduran village, a pregnant woman walked to the *Centro de Salud* and lay down on a cot to one side of the room, her belly rising above her tiny frame like a ripe fruit. While the doctors attended to other patients, the local health aide checked the woman's blood pressure, announcing the result with a sharpness I hadn't heard from her before. I nodded blankly and turned back to the elderly *machetero* telling me about his shoulder pain. Ed, however, strode across the room and tapped expertly on the pregnant woman's right knee with his fingers, his eyes fixed on her quivering lower leg as its oscillations dampened away. He stood up straight and spoke calmly in Spanish to the aide, "This woman needs to go. How quickly can we have the ambulance ready?" The health aide nodded and walked crisply to the front of the building to arrange transportation.

"Clonus," I muttered to myself—the medical term for abnormal deep tendon reflex so exaggerated that the muscles twitch repeatedly, like a pendulum. And then I remembered: exaggerated reflexes in a pregnant woman with even mildly elevated blood pressure signaled pre-eclampsia, a dangerous condition that can lead to maternal seizures and death. In such cases, medicines reduce the danger, but the only cure is prompt delivery of the baby. We handled normal births in the *Centro* and sometimes even in surrounding homes, but this was not a normal birth. She would have to travel to the hospital in La Esperanza, hours up the mountainous dirt road.

I was familiar with pre-eclampsia and its perils from countless calls for a pediatrician to be present at a Caesarian section, but I'd forgotten the simple mechanics of making the diagnosis. Not for the last time, I was grateful for Ed's presence. If I'd been alone, how long would it have taken for me to remember, to recognize the situation? I'd give anything for Ed's breadth of medical knowledge, even more for his skill. If Ed said I needed to see a patient, I didn't doubt him for a moment.

I told him I'd make time before dinner to look in on the kid he was concerned about. Upstairs, in the doctor's quarters, I picked out an unoc-cupied corner bunk in the men's dorm, sliding my bags under the rough wooden bed frame. A medical student dozed in the next bunk while another read silently in the dim light. This had been their home for a week already. They'd share it with me for the week ahead.

I stepped into the bathroom to wash my face. Our presence strains the local water supply. Every trip starts with reminders about water conservation: quick wash-ups, brief showers, the toilet ditty: "if it's yellow, let it mellow." It usually takes me a day or two to get back up to speed, but I remembered this time. A quick splash, once-over with the washcloth, and done.

Back in the common room, Julia, a pediatric resident from Cincinnati, called from the kitchen doorway, "Doctor Volck, you're here." I walked over, gave her a quick hug and asked her how things were going.

"It's been great. I'm really glad I came."

About a year earlier, Julia had asked me about involvement in interna-tional health. I told her then what little I know, and mentioned Shoulder to Shoulder (in Spanish, *Hombro a Hombro*), the organization I'd been work-ing with in rural Honduras for several years. She took it from there, joining the April brigade to Santa Lucia. I was glad to have an experienced pediatric resident with us, especially one so competent.

After chatting lightly about the week's events, she suddenly turned serious. "Did they tell you about our kid with marasmus?" she asked. Ma-rasmus is one of the forms of protein-energy malnutrition. Better known is Kwashiorkor, which gives starving children the bulging bellies, reddish hair and puffy faces seen in news footage from famine-ridden areas in Africa. Marasmus, in contrast, results in total body wasting: twig-like arms, skeletal faces and hollowed bellies straight out of Auschwitz.

The World Health Organization says protein-energy malnutrition affects a quarter of the world's children. WHO reports that 150 million children are underweight, still more stunted in height. Ten million children under five years of age die every year on this planet; half of these suffer from severe malnutrition. Malnourished children who survive still endure pro-longed illnesses and increased vulnerability to disease. Most of the world's severely underfed children live in Asia and Africa. Only 4 percent live in Latin America. Julia was about to introduce me to one of them.

We walked toward the dental clinic and headed downstairs. The room where our patient was staying didn't exist the first time I visited Santa Lucia. Then, there had been a patch of cleared ground marked off with wooden stakes, where men with shovels chipped at the hard, rocky soil. Now it was a large, enclosed space beneath the dental clinic, and had already seen several uses: feeding center, meeting area, patient dormitory. In Honduras, one learns to improvise, use what's available to serve an agreed-upon end.

Downstairs, drawn blinds filtered raking afternoon light onto the tile floor. Idle computers glowed in a corner. Tables, one standing on edge, subdivided the room, one quarter of which was occupied by shadowy figures. As Julia and I silently entered the marked-off area, I saw scattered blankets, a pile of dirty clothes, a half-full plastic water bottle. A woman watched us disinterestedly from a small mattress. There was something artificial and disturbing about the setting, like a family making its home in a department store display window. I'd intruded on something too personal to enter so abruptly, but here I was, expected to sort things out.

My eyes adjusted to the light. I noticed, at last, a black-haired infant leaning against the woman on the mattress. He was small, thin-armed. He could use some calories, but he wasn't nearly as bad as described. When I crouched to examine him, Julia stopped me short, saying, "That's Santos. Roberto is over here." She pointed at a pair of feet and a twisted arm emerging from a cotton blanket. I'd completely missed the patient.

The woman reached over and pulled back the cloth. Partially hidden by a flimsy shred of gingham lay the thinnest human body I'd ever seen, half-heartedly curled into a fetal pose. His legs were bent at the hips and knees. His large, bony feet looked like they'd been grafted onto flesh-covered sticks. He turned slightly to the right, his head flattened to the mattress, left arm bent upward, flicking repeatedly at his patchy scalp, every vein and what little muscle remained in his arms rippling with each stroke of his hand. I lifted the gown. Deep furrows marked the spaces between his ribs. As I was already in a crouch, I waddled around for a better look at his face. His ears looked far too big for the rest of his head. His eyebrows were exuberantly full, but there was no other exuberance about him. A trickle of saliva spilled over red, puffy lips. His face and scalp were scratched. Chunks of thin, lusterless hair were missing. Crusted-over scars filled in the bald patches. But his eyes were irresistible, drawing me into his palace of despair: deep, brown, brooding. When I crouched in line of their gaze, they focused not on me, but somewhere further back, as if by burrowing through my body he might find the source of his misery. I turned away, distressed by his appearance and embarrassed at my silent, clinical stare.

"Where do I begin," I wondered, overmatched by what I saw. Steeling myself with mantras of professionalism, I turned back, feebly attempting an examination. I couldn't think what good I was doing, disturbing him. Still, I listened to his heart and lungs, pressed the slope of his belly. He glared through me, defiant. I turned to his mother. Her name, I learned, was Maria. Her eyes were less intense than her son's: glassier, more distant, as if life had overwhelmed her so many years now that it was no longer worth attending to detail. Though thin by North American standards, she looked reasonably well-fed for a Honduran *campesina*. Her shapeless pink blouse, the top three buttons open, barely concealed her drooping breasts. She had, I supposed, recently nursed Santos. Her hair was pulled back loosely. In her late thirties, she looked fifty. She turned her head when spoken to, and something in her face looked familiar, like a photograph I'd seen in a book. Even in the fullness of her cheeks, there was a frightened, Dust Bowl hollowness. Later, she would make me want to know more. Tonight, I wanted only to leave, and after a brief exchange in my clumsy Spanish, we did.

On our walk back to the dorms, Julia recounted the story so far. She had been part of a field clinic near Santa Rita, ten bone-jarring miles west by dirt road. Late in the afternoon, just before the team packed up for their return, Roberto was carried into the *Centro de Salud*, dirty, urine-drenched, and curled up much as I found him. His sparse hair crawling with lice, he looked dazed, half-dead. Julia gathered important information in the field: Roberto was eight years old and weighed only twenty-seven pounds. His brother, Santos, was also underweight, but not so bad as his brother. Fearing Roberto's death was imminent, the team brought the two boys and their mother back to Santa Lucia in the truck.

Roberto's treatment was well underway by the time I arrived. He'd been rehydrated with IV fluids, the slow process of refeeding begun. A natural inclination is to feed a starving person quickly, making up for lost time with as much food as possible. Such was the approach to survivors of the *Hongerwinter* of 1944, when the collapsing Nazi occupation and severe cold reduced the Dutch to eating tulip bulbs. Following the Allied liberation, those fed aggressively did poorly. Many died of what's now known as refeeding syndrome. The lesson learned was that the starved body is even more fragile than it appears. Starving patients can be killed with the kindness of food. But Roberto took poorly even the small amounts of mineral-rich food we permitted him. His weight was up, but that was surely from fluid replacement. If Roberto was going to survive, we had to find a way for him to eat.

That evening, after dinner, the doctors gathered to talk over the brigade's first week in Honduras. Average acuity of illness—a measure of the urgency of patient complaints—continued its slow decrease from previous years—a trend we attributed to the presence of a permanently staffed clinic. Since the arrival of Shoulder to Shoulder in Santa Lucia, many longstanding conditions had been addressed and, by degrees, controlled. Compared to field clinics in outlying villages, where we treated many tropical conditions no longer seen in North America, patient visits in Santa Lucia increasingly resembled those at home. Nutritional deficiencies and other preventable illnesses had given way to diabetes, high blood pressure, and cardiovascular disease. Even in the few years I had been coming to Santa Lucia, there were clear improvements in living conditions, perhaps due less to the clinic than to family members emigrating to the United States and sending needed cash back home.

Improved living conditions brought a corresponding rise in expectations, now sorely challenged by the discovery of a severely malnourished child. Such things were no longer taken for granted in this part of the country, yet here Roberto was. He presented a similar challenge to the medical team, who were determined to bring him through this crisis and restore him to something like health. Just how remained a mystery.

It was Jim, our dentist, who first called attention to Roberto's teeth. Most were rotten and infected, presenting a double threat. Severe decay made eating painful, which explained at least some of Roberto's reluctance to eat. Worse still, starvation crippled his ability to fight off infection. Bacteria from a tooth abscess might easily invade his bloodstream and seed his heart, his lungs, his brain. Roberto's toothaches were more than an inconvenience. They threatened his life. In a hastily called conference of doctors and dentists, we decided to remove all Roberto's infected teeth in two stages: right side first, then left. Jim worried aloud that the stress of extraction might be enough to kill Roberto, even if leaving his teeth in place seemed certain death: "He's so sick, and I don't want to be the one who kills him." His bluntness forced us to think harder. This was strange territory for most of us, and we agreed on a cautious approach. Plans were made to tackle part one the following day. In preparation, Julia and Liz, another pediatric resident, deloused Roberto again. They gowned and gloved, anticipating another explosion of vermin fleeing his body, much as Julia witnessed with his first treatment. Julia visibly enjoyed cleaning up her patient and even called to the medical students, "Anyone who wants to see lice in all life stages, come quick!" After shampooing his hair, they cut most of it off.

Debbie, Jim's wife and dental assistant, prepared Roberto for the extractions, visiting him as often as she could. "I wanted to make some sense of why this was happening to him—and to other children in the world," she later told me. She, too, was drawn in by Roberto's brown eyes: "They were almost like God telling me, 'We have to do something here.'" Debbie sat with Roberto and his mother, touching him, holding him, talking through an interpreter to the mother who, as several of us noted, looked remarkably detached for the mother of a gravely ill child.

"I don't think this child has been touched," Debbie told me. "No one's stroked him, held his head. I don't think these kids have gotten that. When I do it, he seems to like it." In an effort not to judge Roberto's mother too harshly, Debbie tried to learn more from clinic workers and villagers from Santa Rita. Their stories were contradictory. Some of Maria's neighbors claimed she was a terrible mother, perhaps mentally ill. They wanted little to do with her. A man from the clinic committee later challenged one of the neighbors on this, telling her to look in on the kids even if she didn't like Maria. Some claimed Maria's husband—whom I had yet to meet—drank away what little money the family had. Others said he was as good a father as anyone could be in such desperate conditions. We had no way to decide which accounts to trust, which to discount.

Debbie and others from the clinic started preparing Roberto's mother for an eventual return home. They showed her how to feed Roberto pureed foods, one spoonful at a time. The clinic staff soon realized Maria had no experience keeping a room clean. Later, when we saw the one room family house, its uneven dirt floor and porous walls through which dogs and chickens scurried, it was clear why. Someone at the clinic gave Maria a broom, showed how to tidy up her room, and told her she was to continue doing so as long as they stayed. She'd have to have to learn new skills if Roberto was going to live and, the thinking went, cleanliness was a good place to start.

* * * *

When I think back on those first days with Roberto, conversations among the medical team at the time mix with those I know came later, after we returned north, still burdened by our encounter with Roberto. We meet each other on occasion, in a hospital hallway or in church, sometimes speaking his name, as if to reassure ourselves the conversation hasn't ended. It's as if we're still lingering after dinner outside the clinic in Santa Lucia, sipping coffee, trying to make sense of the day's events while the kitchen staff washes the plates:

Debbie: *"Maria says she was abandoned by her parents at sixteen. I can't imagine what she understood of life at sixteen. And this husband—he's her second—isn't Roberto's father. I'm pretty sure Roberto is Maria's tenth child.*

Even she loses track when she goes through all the names. Santos followed real soon afterward, and she's pregnant again by this husband.

"It's hard to figure out when Roberto got so ill. Maria says Roberto was doing well until he came down with diarrhea, that it just wouldn't go away. This was about six months before we met. Maria says he was able to walk before that, and all his weakness started then."

Me: "Diarrhea is a big problem in developing countries, but the timing here doesn't make sense. Roberto's so thin, you know, so short. His malnutrition must have started quite early. Maybe a recent diarrhea episode made things worse, but he hasn't been getting enough calories for years.

"He's got a lot of what we call 'soft signs,' physical findings which, by themselves, don't necessarily make a diagnosis, though they suggest Roberto was never quite right. His hairline is low enough to blend with his eyebrows, and the hair on the back of his neck keeps going all the way down to his shoulders. Look at the size of his ears, the coarseness of his face and those tiny, curved fifth fingers. We call that finger bit 'clinodactyly.' You know, taken as a whole, I'd guess he's got some congenital syndrome—something we haven't diagnosed yet—an inborn problem that stunted him intellectually. Perhaps physically, too. In any case, his heel cords—his Achilles' tendons—are short and tight. He hasn't walked in months, if ever. "

Jim: "I don't think he was ever right. With all those mouths to feed, he just never got to the table in time. When Santos came along, Roberto was left out. I don't think it was because they didn't care. They just didn't have enough."

Liz, a first-year pediatric resident: "I wonder how we must look to Roberto's mother. Even though kids in the States may go to bed hungry, they aren't this sick with malnutrition. I mean, so here we are, running in and out of the room, taking pictures, asking questions, acting all panicked, and she's just sitting there smiling as if nothing's happening. We're in emergency caretaking mode, and her response doesn't make sense. We aren't going to show her the same deference, the same respect we might show a mother back home. We end up blaming her, like she gave up on him. But Santos is sick, too. I mean, who was she supposed to pick?

"I've seen malnourished kids before, in Kenya, but Roberto is worse than any single child I can remember. Something went seriously wrong, sometime in his short life. So why is it so hard to get a coherent story? Nothing quite adds up to explain it all. Is it lack of trust? No time? Are we stuck with a bad translation? Or are all the stories part of the truth and we have to figure out the best way to make sense of them all?"

Liz was right. In the United States, we review medical records, those alleg-
edly objective documents doctors fill with crumbs of information and mold
into a coherent story. In Santa Lucia, we kept trying to cobble one story out
of several, and we couldn't make everything fit. We'd wandered into strange
country without a map, each of us desperately trying to remember the way
back home, but the memories never agreed. Something had to go, but how
were we to know which memories were correct and crucial, which illusory
or irrelevant? The more we learned, the more lost we felt.

* * * *

The morning Roberto lost his teeth, the doctors were busy with medical patients. I visited the dental clinic just before Jim and Debbie started. Roberto
lay on a dental chair, his limbs splayed about his frail and spindly torso.
Debbie had taken great care to make him comfortable, even cozy. A blanket
covered him. The room was bright with sunlight. Posters about dental care
and pictures of sunny tropical locations hung on the walls.

"How's the patient?" I asked.

"Doing all right, aren't you Roberto?" Debbie said with a motherly
turn of her head.

I'd seen Jim and Debbie work in another Honduran village two years
earlier, pulling rotten teeth for hours in a dimly lit cinder block clinic. The
two of them were visibly grateful to serve this way. They shook their heads
at injustice and questioned administrative foolishness, but I'd never heard
either one complain. I knew they would handle today's procedure, and I
headed back to the clinic.

Roberto came through wonderfully, better than anyone suspected. After a brief recovery, he ate a little and slept reasonably well that night. He was
getting stronger, and not just physically. "What a stinker he can be," Debbie
said, "He was mad at us when we pulled his teeth, you could tell that, but
he also seemed to get that we were doing our best to help. He liked being in
recovery with the fan blowing on him, being washed up, being taken care of
in ways that were new to him. He was feeling better, and he was—to me—
just beautiful. Everybody's own kids are the most beautiful child, I know,
but right then, he was the most beautiful child in the world, a gift to me."

Debbie and Roberto were together quite often, and her smile—radiant
enough to hide the sorrow in her eyes—was one of gratitude. Alone among
the *Norteamericanos,* Debbie broke through the cultural divides and forged
emotional links. Julia was Roberto's primary doctor, and loved Roberto

every bit as much and just as fiercely, but she had to remain his physician, constantly reassessing the patient before her. Debbie had the freedom to simply be with him. I watched Debbie walk into the room, almost singing her greeting, and Roberto burst into smiles, followed her with his eyes, brightened at her voice. The shadowy place still smelled of old, dirty clothes and sweat, but it seemed brighter, cooler when they were together. While recovering from the second set of extractions in the dental clinic, Roberto began to play with Debbie. His rotten teeth lay in a metal basin. Debbie sponged blood from his lips. Lounging before a fan, Roberto luxuriated in friendly company. They looked at each other while Debbie stroked his face, but every time she turned to speak to someone in the busy clinic, Roberto moaned, desperate to regain her attention. She turned back, smile, and they began again. "He wanted my attention, all of it," Debbie explained later, "and he turned that into a game."

I'd like to imagine a similar connection would arise between any two people thrown together in such circumstances, but Roberto and Debbie weren't "any two people." They flourished together, two persons folded into a single membership. Debbie and Roberto's visible affection was infectious, and I caught the germ myself. I wanted to understand how he'd gotten so sick. I wanted him to get better.

It was here that we, as a group, let fantasy overtake reality. Some of the medical team began to talk about things we could do to rescue Roberto and his family. We might do a thorough "needs assessment" of his house, determine what could be corrected, offer a steady supply of food, guarantee clean, drinkable water. Some imagined the state of Roberto's home, which turned out, in the end, to be worse than we supposed. Some suggested Roberto could be flown back to the States for adequate nutrition, a full developmental and medical evaluation, and comprehensive treatment, but others asked in return why we would select this family for "rescue" and not another. I considered taking a small tissue sample from Roberto back to the States, perhaps to definitively diagnose his condition. As an organization, Shoulder to Shoulder has, on occasion, taken extraordinary steps for single patients and families, but the guiding principle of the effort is communal action. Was this what the Hondurans wanted? How would flying Roberto north improve things? Were he ill from a correctable heart defect or treatable injury, there was hope in such plans. But Roberto was, as far as we could tell, beyond curing. Even an exact diagnosis was unlikely to help, however intellectually satisfying it would be to know what my patient had. Roberto's "treatment options" were few. We were coming to grips with the crucial difference between curing and caring. We were learning how to care when cure is impossible.

Later, back in the States, Debbie reflected on the assumptions of control dominating most of our talk about rescuing Roberto: "I don't know
what they thought they were going to do. As much as I care about Roberto,
it didn't make any sense to take him away from everything he's ever known
just to satisfy us. It's hard for me to say but, while I know I'll be sad when I
learn that Roberto has died—sad especially because I didn't get to see him
one more time—I won't be sad for him. I know he's never going to grow up
to be a man or a father. I just want what life he has left to be as good as it can
be where he is."

That's a sort of letting go North Americans find hard to embrace, a letting
go Honduras can teach someone who brings the right practice of attention.
North Americans like stories that move in an orderly way, flying straight
from bowstring to target, where the tip buries itself into the bullseye with a
satisfying "thunk." Hondurans expect interrupted tales, taking sudden turns
or meandering off like a mountain road, circling back only when the other
trail gives out. Maybe that's another habit of attention—holding one story in
suspense while another plays out. This is a Honduran story.

Tuesday evening, after what Ed called his favorite Honduran meal—
tortillas, refried beans and *crema*, a cheesy sour cream sauce—I was looking forward to sitting down on the front steps of the dormitory. I find the
Honduran dusk too steamy for ambitious physical effort, but perfect for
digesting a meal or reading a good book. I planned to do both, though I
gathered from the voices rising from below that something was going on in
the clinic. This, however, wasn't my night on call. I planned to relax. A few
minutes later, one of the attendings, an Emergency Medicine doc I never
hit it off with, mentioned, to no one particular, that a sick kid had arrived
downstairs. I sank further behind my book, waiting for someone to actually
tell me I was needed, but curiosity and conscience got the best of me. I
was the only board certified pediatrician present. If there really was a sick
kid—by no means certain, since even good doctors can misread the signs of
severe illness in children—I had better go look. If the child was fine, I could
get back to reading.

The clinic downstairs was nearly empty, but worried voices came from
the examining room at the end of the hallway. I entered. On the table to
the left of the doorway lay a boy, perhaps a year old, looking gravely ill, his
breaths coming in fast shallow gasps, his chest working hard with each res-
piration. His face was nearly as pale as the white cinder block walls, but the
rest of his skin was smeared with a green, slimy paste. His eyes were glassy,
rolled upward, their whiteness looking like death. This would not be quick.

The nursing student had taken a quick set of vital signs: pulse 200, temperature 107 degrees Fahrenheit. I pressed my fingers against his neck to check a carotid pulse: too fast to count. A pulse of 200 was probably correct, but his skin, though hot to touch, did not suggest a temperature so dangerously high. I asked where she'd put the thermometer.

"Axillary," she said, meaning under the arm.

"Can we get a rectal temp, please?" Among the very few things I do well in emergency situations is maintain an appearance of calm. It's all show, of course. Underneath my studied politeness, I'm struggling, wondering what to do next. I suspect I learned some of that from the director of the intensive care unit where I trained during residency. An enormous man, brilliant and capable, he let the medical team know things were going well with a flow of jokes and insults. Once he assumed a mask of politeness, though, something was wrong: one of us, we knew, had screwed up badly. From him, I learned to keep a light touch in dire circumstances. Later, the nurses in the Indian Health Service used to ask me to run their mock codes—practices runs for life or death emergencies—because I "didn't yell at them." It seemed a strange way to pick a mentor. I felt particularly out of my depth in true emergencies, but had ample opportunity to work on demeanor and get the drill down: the rubrics of responding to a child near death. It was precisely those rubrics I had to fall back upon here. There's something reassuring in practiced habits, even in the midst of panic.

"Anyone know a history?" I asked.

"He was seen in clinic earlier today and sent home. Something about fever and diarrhea."

Just then, Liz and Julia arrived. I was grateful for the additional help. There was much to do. The rectal temperature came back as 104, a more likely figure than 107, but still very high. Someone brought us a vial labeled "antipyretic," a Honduran medicine that the clinic used to treat high fevers. It could only be given by injection. Considering this child's grim appearance of clouded consciousness, we had no alternative for lowering his fever, so we injected the medicine into his thigh after cleaning away the greenish slime. He barely whimpered.

In an emergency, we return to the ABCs: airway, breathing, circulation. The child—whose name, we came to learn was Jenrry, pronounced like Eliza Doolittle's "'enry 'iggins," but with a Latin trill to the double r—had maintained his airway and breathing so far, as a brief listen to his chest with the stethoscope quickly verified. It was clear, however, that he could not keep breathing this fast for long. He would tire soon, unable to provide sufficient oxygen and blow off enough carbon dioxide to meet his body's demands. Lacking tools to measure oxygen in his blood, we offered a nasal cannula, a clear plastic tube with one tiny prong for each nostril, connected on the other end to an oxygen tank. That would help for a short while we considered Jenrry's circulation.

We needed to obtain IV access somewhere, give this child fluids, and get his heart rate down or all the oxygen in the world wouldn't help. Julia and Liz began poking at Jenrry's arms, trying to place an IV, but with no success. They toweled away more green, hunting for the bluish tint of a likely vein. I announced a five-minute maximum to search for regular IV access before we would be forced to try something less conventional. Five minutes passed quickly. We decided to try an intraosseous line, a needle placed straight into the bone.

In young children, there is enough space in the marrow of tibia—"the shin bone"—to place a thick needle and supply fluid and medicines. Nowadays there are drills designed specifically for placing intraosseous lines, but no such device existed at that time and not in Honduras. Unable to find a proper "IO needle" in the clinic, we opened a sterile lumbar puncture kit for the stiff needle used in spinal taps. It would have to do. Julia had never placed an IO line before and was eager to try. I talked her through the procedure, showing her where to place the tip, the angle at which to proceed, the slight twisting motion to make as she drove the tip through the bone itself. I noted with increasing concern that, all the while we were pressing a needle into Jenrry's shin, he barely responded to the pain we caused him.

"Keep pressing until you feel the 'pop,'" I said.

"There it is," she said.

"Good. Take out the stylet and we'll hook it up to some fluids."

We twisted an IV line onto the needle hub and turned the fluid wide open. Nothing happened. No fluid was moving. I pressed on the IV bag to give it some force. Nothing again. We turned the needle, pushing it back and forward. Still nothing. This was not going well. If we couldn't quickly find a way to give our patient fluids, he would surely die.

"Should we try another?" Julia asked.

"Maybe," I said, not entirely sure if anything we were doing would keep this child from dying while we watched. Someone remembered one of the attending physicians—named Jim, just like our dentist—worked as an anesthesiologist back in the States. A doctor with skill at finding IV access in the most difficult of situations would do better than any of us.

He was down in a moment. We told him the situation and he immediately began searching along Jenrry's neck. An external jugular line, placed in the large vein of the neck, would give us the access we needed, but with a host of risks. The anatomy is a little scary, so close to the large arteries supplying blood to the brain. If he was successful, the challenge would soon come of keeping a child from dislodging the catheter with sudden neck movements or, if he grew more alert, by grabbing at the line and pulling it out. We'd deal with that later. Right now we needed a line—any line. In minutes Jim was taping a catheter in place, covering the plastic with thick layers of gauze. Saline was already running, filling Jenrry's vessels with what he most needed. Jim seemed to shrug off his success as routine, but the pediatricians were grateful, loudly breathing sighs of relief and permitting ourselves a brief reassurance that this might, after all, turn out well.

With an IV running and Jenrry's vital signs stabilizing, we reentered familiar territory, a mental location where the routine was known, where the expected should happen. We reexamined the patient, noting aloud findings what I had quickly passed over before: pupils narrowed to black pinpoints, diminished muscle tone in arms and legs, minimal response to pain, persistent watery diarrhea and the still mysterious coating of green on his skin. We speculated what might be causing such findings: infection to be sure, given the presentation of fever and shock, but the tiny pupils and bizarrely elevated vital signs suggested toxic ingestion—a mistake in medication or accidental poisoning. And what was all this green? Diarrhea? Something he'd fallen into? We would give him antibiotics to cover any infection, but we'd need more information to help sort out the possible matter of poisoning.

Julia and Liz went to speak to the family: a toothless, shrunken grandmother in a green dress standing with a much younger woman and boy in the hallway. After I tidied up and calculated Jenrry's first antibiotic dose, the two residents returned with the story as they had heard it. The elderly woman was indeed Jenrry's grandmother; the other two Jenrry's teenage aunt and pre-teen brother. Jenrry's mother had died in childbirth, approximately a year ago. Where Jenrry's father was, we never learned.

The grandmother confirmed that this was the child seen earlier in the day in clinic. He'd fallen ill with diarrhea and fever but, at the time of his visit, was attentive, even playful, in between sips of milk. Julia had seen him at that visit. Reassured that he was not dehydrated, she sent him home with advice on giving fluids and managing fever. This was, after all, a common enough complaint in Honduras as well as the United States.

After the clinic visit, however, Jenrry's grandmother took him to a local traditional healer, who gave him nothing by mouth, but instead rubbed a mixture of alcohol and *ruta,* a local plant, into Jenrry's skin. As best we could determine, the plant was a relative of the tomato, placing it in the same botanical family as nightshade, and raising interesting possible explanations for Jenrry's condition. First of all, the green slime was likely part of the healer's salve. Second, we knew that many nightshade plants contain highly potent alkaloids—plant-derived pharmacologic substances—with effects often consistent with "anticholinergic syndrome": hallucinations or clouded consciousness, racing pulse, fever, dry mucous membranes and flushing of the skin. Some of these fit Jenrry, but unfortunately for us, anticholinergic effects also include large pupils, not small. Could a combination of alkaloids have passed through his skin to explain what we were seeing? Perhaps there was more to *ruta* or this salve than we knew. In any case, the family had decided to bring Jenrry back to us when he turned for the worse, his alertness fading into stupor, his diarrhea accelerating with his pulse.

Not much to go on, we agreed, but it we at least had a place to start. Together, we reassessed the patient. Still unresponsive even though his heart rate and capillary refill had improved, we knew that in the mountains of Honduras there was little hope of identifying or definitively treating a serious toxic ingestion. We'd already tried to run a blood sample on the chemistry machine in the lab, hoping for a more precise guide to our fluid management, but the results were bizarre. The machine clearly wasn't working properly. We would do our best with what we had, and we had made some progress already. Before we had a chance to pat ourselves on the back, however, I saw something new and ominous: Jenrry's arms were stiffening, extended straight outward in what is called decerebrate posturing, suggesting injury to the brain. For the second time that night, I feared our patient was dying.

The posturing soon stopped, although we did see occasional eye fluttering and stiffening of his right arm, suggestive of seizures. These too, however, ceased. We called the family to sit with him. The grandmother and sister stepped into the room, looking uncomfortable, out of their element, but anxious to see and touch Jenrry. They were careful with him, studiously gentle, as if sudden movement would break him. The grandmother quietly moaned but said nothing. They looked grave, said they had no questions for us, and turned to find seats against the opposite wall.

His antibiotics given, his vital signs much improved, and his neurologic exam a bit more stable—if not exactly reassuring—Liz, Julia and I made plans for Jenrry's care overnight. Liz volunteered for the first shift, and I made sure she was comfortable with the tasks ahead of her. I went to bed, but slept fitfully, awakening often, puzzling over the mystery of our patient, wondering how many crucial details I had missed.

Liz remembers the night as one of dread, tempered by the busyness of the tasks assigned her. She gave IV antibiotics, changed Jenrry's soupy yellow diapers, and tried without success to get Jenrry's sister to lie down and sleep. The two of them sat at the bedside, saying almost nothing, staring at the child who had brought them together. Overnight, they each attended to him according to their talents, the way a servant stands by, ready to assist. At 2:30 a.m., Jenrry was due for another injection of "antipyretic," his temperature hovering above the 100 F mark. With this injection into his thigh, though, Jenrry cried lustily, the torment of his past several hours set free at last. Jenrry's sister rushed to care for him, but Liz watched through her tears with wonder, encouraged by this display that the boy might actually pull through.

By morning's light, we had a sleeping but visibly improved patient and a host of medical decisions waiting to be made. Diagnostic resources in Santa Lucia were even more limited than our therapies. We had a broken blood chemistry analyzer; no means to culture spinal fluid, blood, or urine for evidence of bacterial infection; and no CT scanner. The portable X-Ray machine looked like a Renaissance torture device and produced films of dubious quality.

For therapy, we had a small cache of Ceftriaxone, an injectable antibiotic purchased in the States with Shoulder to Shoulder money and carried in our suitcases on the way down. This was meant to supply the clinic for months. If we dosed Jenrry with enough to treat possible meningitis—as we would do back home in the absence of reliable spinal fluid cultures—we'd empty the pharmacy shelf and still run short. We had neither sufficient money nor a source from which to obtain more Ceftriaxone in Honduras. Liz acidly noted that in the Emergency Room in Cincinnati, Ceftriaxone flows like water. For Jenrry in Santa Lucia, it was more precious than drinkable water—and harder to come by.

After speaking with Marvin, one of our Honduran doctors, who ruled out the possibility of getting any more Ceftriaxone to the clinic in the time needed, we decided on a compromise course: slightly shorter in total number of days, and at doses to cover for serious infection, but not for meningitis. We pretended this was a calculated risk, but there was little real calculation in anything we were doing now. Everything now was compromise and guesswork, an improvised course of action through which carefully learned habits formed in the technologically rich North were adapted to local circumstances.

Throughout our dithering and discussion, Jenrry's grandmother and sister looked after the boy. Jenrry's sister seemed forever occupied with housekeeping tasks while the grandmother—always in the dark green dress she refused to change despite our frequent offers of clean clothes—flashed a toothless grin as Jenrry sucked at a bottle. They were beautiful together: an elderly woman, her brown face furrowed deeply as she pondered her grandson; the ill child whose eyes cleared and brightened as he grew stronger.

Sometimes I'd walk into the room and find the grandmother half sitting, half reclining on the exam table, a folded towel covering the top of her head in an outlandish bonnet, and she'd just be looking silently at this boy. She kept telling us how grateful she was for the things we had done, for saving her grandson, comments we politely accepted before returning to work.

In truth, though, Jenrry still worried us. He improved vastly in the first twenty-four hours after his nighttime arrival, but then his recovery's trajectory leveled. He was more alert, even smiling at times, his eyes like burning anthracite; but his muscle tone remained disappointingly floppy. His fevers were gone, but he still had episodes of diarrhea. He was better—but not all better—and the North Americans were quickly approaching the end of our stay in Santa Lucia. Had we been in the States, we would not only be planning a longer course of antibiotic therapy, but also a thorough rehabilitative medicine and physical therapy evaluation, to determine what services the family might need after discharge. None of that would happen here. We saved Jenrry's life, but would he survive when we left? There would be no visiting nurse, no early intervention services, no school-based therapy program. When we left Santa Lucia, the Honduran doctors would come along, seeing us to the airport and taking a well-earned vacation after the chaos of welcoming thirty guests to their workplace for two weeks. We needed to find a way for Jenrry to make it in his home.

The same, we knew, went for Roberto.

* * * *

Roberto ate better without his rotting teeth. He felt better, too. He no longer telegraphed misery with every movement. He smiled more often, even when Debbie wasn't present. With a close-cropped haircut, he looked less bedraggled, more like boys his age, but we knew he wasn't cured. What we'd done in our short time together was halt his slide toward death by starvation. Any real change in the course of his life depended on his family's response when he returned home. Encouraging basic housekeeping skills for Maria became more urgent. Roberto's mother, we knew, would be the key to Roberto's course once home.

But Roberto's room began to stink. Soap and water were readily available but rarely used. Dirty diapers stewed in place before being changed. Extra visits to Roberto and his family, which once the doctors and students made at whim, soon stopped. Medical personnel now entered only when absolutely necessary. When the family finally left, staff workers thoroughly sprayed down the room before using it again.

Janina Galler, a Boston University psychiatrist and public health researcher, studied children on the island of Barbados who were severely malnourished in their first year of life. In her many years observing and testing the survivors, Galler traced the legacy of developmental and behavioral disorders that follow not having enough to eat as an infant. She also documented troubling effects of maternal depression upon early child development. Whether any of this data could be appropriately applied to Roberto, whose starvation occurred at a later age than the Barbadians Galler follows, is uncertain, but the mysterious dance of mother and child had clearly been disrupted in Roberto's and Maria's case. How else could one explain why Debbie, at least for the time we had known him, was a better mother to Roberto than Maria could be?

There were compelling reasons to believe that Roberto's delays were, at least in part, consequences of a congenital condition, but he grew worse with Santos's arrival. Absent growth charts and periodic measurements, we couldn't pinpoint the key moment or moments in Roberto's decline. How large a role Roberto's recent struggle for calories played in his current problems was also beyond our ability to determine. So we asked other questions, like: "What can we do to help Maria?" meaning for the most part, "How can we help Maria help her sons?" Only after we saw the house in which she raised her children did we begin to appreciate the obstacles Maria faced. Several of us wondered how she'd managed to help Roberto survive even this long.

Plans were assembled for Roberto's return, a crude venture compared to the complex discharge rituals in American hospitals. The day before the brigade was scheduled to pull out of Santa Lucia, as we readied a pair of pickup trucks to take Roberto back to Santa Rita, Roberto's stepfather appeared suddenly in clinic. He was a wiry man, thinner than Maria, with a black moustache and a narrow face topped by a gray cowboy hat. His eyes were dark, expressive, and hollow, like Roberto's. He stared silently at our disorderly preparations, hands hidden in the pockets of his jeans, his thick eyebrows raised in mild astonishment. Debbie helped Maria, Santos, and Roberto into the truck cabin. Later, she told me about the ride in the cabin with the family, "Roberto got real somber, and stopped making eye contact. No more smiles the whole trip. It felt like we were going to a funeral for kids who were still alive. Roberto had gotten a little better while he was with us and now we were taking him back to where he'd gotten so sick in the first place. I didn't expect he would live very long."

Outside Santa Rita—less a town than a few buildings that look like they accidentally strayed together and would soon disperse—our sad caravan pulled off the road and parked where the mountain rose sharply before us. Maria, her husband and two kids climbed out immediately and waited while the gringos collected their gear and tightened laces on expensive hiking boots. Once ready, we started up the footpath, Maria—pregnant and wearing plastic flip-flops—charging ahead in the lead, a gaggle of Americans huffing behind her. It was dry season, and the corn harvest was in. Withered stalks stood in tattered formation. Even the trees looked weary and dry.

We straddled a crumbling stone wall, negotiated a few switchbacks, and climbed up through the family's *milpa*, a picked-over corn patch tumbling down the unterraced slope. I stumbled several times trying to keep Maria's pace. Some of Roberto's brothers and sisters saw us coming, their cries of excitement cheering those of us already tiring from the ascent.

Cresting the ridge, we found a small clearing with a stirring view of the Salvadoran mountains to the south. Everything else about the place was dispiriting. The house—a one room hut—stood in the center. Adobe walls crumbled under a roof of tile and wood. There was no floor save well-compressed dirt, no doors to close. A scrawny pig chased three nearly featherless chickens into the house while a hungry-looking dog panted silently at the open doorway. A plastic drinking cup hung by a string from a forked log near the outdoor bread oven. On the limbs of a short, naked tree nearby hung several empty plastic containers, their faded and peeling labels warning in Spanish of the toxic effects of herbicide.

We entered the house. A small wood stove smoldered in the corner. Smoke stung my eyes. The interior wall was reinforced with plywood. A stone *metate*, worn smooth from years of making meal from corn, stood next to a hand-operated food grinder. A low bench and table were laden with pitchers and plates. Maria carried her son to the far side of the rear doorway and placed him on a small bed frame strung with a raffia-like fiber. On this tiny bed—and on the surrounding floor—nine people slept. Julia and Liz presented the family with a hammock and looked about for a place to string it up. Roberto, at least, would have someplace other than the floor to sit. We also brought a small amount of food to be pureed for Roberto as well as some plastic bins and basins.

Roberto's brother, Jose, who looked about twelve or thirteen, offered to show us the family's source of water. We headed out back, following another footpath to a hollow in the mountain face. We could smell water, and occasionally glimpsed a trickle below us, but we walked a quarter mile before spying an elderly woman ankle deep in a small, rocky pool. She held two gourds, pouring water over her head with one. This water, Jose told us, was used for cooking and bathing. We walked further upstream, finding another, even smaller natural basin that served as the family's drinking water source. I counted two other houses further up the slope and assumed there were more I couldn't see. Waste from above would contaminate everything downstream, including the small stagnant pool before us. We made plans to bring one of the project's locally made water purification devices here. Where would it go? Who, besides Roberto's family, would use it? And what *did* the village think about all this? Shoulder to Shoulder relies on community involvement and direction rather than going around posing as the smart gringos with an answer to every problem. The water issue would take some thinking. More importantly, it required the community choosing to do something about it.

We returned to the hut. Mondardo, a member of the Santa Lucia clinic board, was sitting on an outside bench, talking earnestly with Roberto's stepfather. Someone pointed out two or three empty beer cans littering the slope. Debbie, who had stayed behind at the hut while we walked to the water source, said one of Roberto's older brothers, relatively well groomed and smelling of aftershave, had stopped by to get some food. One of the interpreters stopped him, saying he should be leaving food, not taking it. He was sixteen—a man now—and he needed to care for the rest of the family.

Suddenly, Mondardo and the stepfather were done with their conference and everyone stepped inside the hut. Roberto lay on the bed, looking bewildered and sad. Santos sat next to him, in one of the plastic basins, raising his thick eyebrows and trying to raise a smile. One of the girls who, we were told, stayed home and helped Maria with the children rather than go to school, stood nearby. She watched the boys while the adults were busy. Someone discreetly slipped her cash for school. Mondardo addressed us as a group. He said a short prayer for the family and their continued safety and health. We said our goodbyes to Roberto and left.

We kept a grim silence on our walk back to the truck. Debbie's funeral image felt exactly right, each of us certain we'd seen Roberto for the last time. Our shared experiences with Roberto and Jenrry over the past week had reminded me the practice of "attending" isn't merely to listen or pay attention, but also to be present, to serve, to accompany. What we'd just done looked and felt like abandonment.

Liz shared her thoughts after that silent march: "How, I wondered, could anyone make things work in that place? How could you feed anybody there? Everything is so far away: water, food, the road. What time did Roberto's mother have to wake up in the morning to get anything done: making breakfast, tending the corn, hauling water? And if you end up bathing in your own stagnant water source, no wonder you're always dirty and smelly. If I'd been put in that situation as a teenager, I know I'd fail."

Debbie remembers thinking, "No wonder she doesn't use a broom. What's the point of sweeping?"

Mostly, though, Debbie was silent and kept to herself, looking like a mother mourning a lost child. All of us were sad, but saying goodbye to Roberto fell hardest on her. No one spoke on the ride back to Santa Lucia.

Once there, though, we concerned ourselves with preparations our own departure. There was also the matter of Jenrry to settle. The boy continued to make slow progress toward what we hoped would be full recovery. The IV was out of his neck and he now turned his head freely, lighting up the room with his smile. Yet he wasn't back to normal—too weak and floppy for his age, not at all like the vibrant child his family described before the illness. He was able to drink and eat, but his stools, once watery, had turned into something like the green slime he'd been covered with upon arrival. We were still in the morass we'd entered once our expensive drugs and well-practiced drills pulled him back from death. Why wasn't his body—why wasn't he—cooperating?

I revisited the pharmacy shelves to count boxes of Cextriaxone. We'd already pillaged the supply. There was little left for the clinic to use until the next North American brigade. Even if we had more, we still had no idea what we were treating. We had no cultures to rule out bacterial infection, no lab tests pointing the way towards rational, high-tech therapy. Perhaps Jenrry was getting better despite our treatment. We had no way of knowing where we were. There was a hospital in La Esperanza, four hours back up the road, a town through which we would pass on our way back to the airport and home, but there was little they could do there that we weren't already doing in Santa Lucia. There was even a children's hospital in Tegucigalpa, the capital, but no money to fund the kind of rehabilitative care Jenrry would need. Jenrry would have to go home and recover with his family.

Learning to trust the body is hard for doctors trained to master the flesh. Powerful tools and miraculous technology impoverish a physician's understanding of the body's powers and limits. So used to my scientific weaponry, of coaxing the body towards whatever we choose to call health, I felt naked, publicly unmasked, deprived of my bag of medical tricks. We would have to trust Jenrry, his body, his family. We had no choice.

Liz stayed up late with Jenrry and his sister, showing her how to mix up formula and bottles of oral rehydration solution to be used at home. She filled a bag with oral antibiotics, medicines for fever, and a few small blankets. The family lived well off the main road, far up the hills. A clinic worker offered to drive them home. It was already dark and all the North Americans were busy. There would be no farewell team as there'd been with Roberto.

I watched as Jenrry's grandmother and sister climbed into the truck, once again startled at the spryness of Honduran elders. Liz placed Jenrry carefully on his grandmother's lap, loose stool dripping from his cloth diaper. I waved, said goodbye. Liz lingered alongside until the truck was ready to move, looking intently at the boy who lived because we had been there, and who was going home. The truck began inching toward the gate. Liz turned away, not letting them see her tears.

* * * *

The bus ride from Santa Lucia was uneventful. While most of the brigade left for the States from Tegucigalpa—a bleak, dispiriting Central American capital—I headed to Guatemala for an international health conference. Guatemala's capital is no prize either: a sprawling octopus groping into the hills; a morass of poverty, random murder and warring gangs, yet more vibrant, even in its squalor, than Tegucigalpa. The bus route from Guatemala City to Antigua, home to the conference, wound through green hillsides unlike anything I'd seen in Honduras. In Antigua, I checked into a sixteenth-century house turned hotel. After my cramped quarters in Santa Lucia, the room seemed huge: Spanish colonial furniture, a bathroom, television, bottled water.

Antigua hovers between times, cultures, and economies. Crumbling colonial churches stand near plazas where consumer-savvy Mayan peasants peddle wares. Rich Northern professionals map out vacations in upscale hotels near ruined monasteries. Antigua stands on treacherous ground, its surroundings unstable, volcanically active. Once the colonial capital, it was rebuilt after serial earthquakes until the government decamped for less volatile land. I did a double take one morning as I left the conference site: a nearby volcano spewed dark gray ash skyward. Sidewalk peddlers paid no attention, eagerly displaying wares to passing gringos. No one seemed alarmed. In an alley lined with restaurants and shops, I found an Internet café and gushed in an email to my daughter about the beauty of her native country, how different everything appeared now that that long and terrible Guatemalan civil war—a war set in motion by North American plans to "fix" Guatemala through a military coup—was over. Scars of war are hidden from tourists. The locals know what happened on the terraced hills, but keep their silence. If you want to see what war did to Guatemala, look in the eyes. Suffering lingers there in those who have no choice but to endure.

In between conference sessions, I traveled the countryside, visiting a mission hospital, housing and reforestation projects, and a cooperative business managed by war widows. With so much to see and think about, I tried not to mull over Roberto and Jenrry, but they lingered, surfacing at night as I pulled up the covers in the chill Guatemalan darkness. My mind raced. "How could I change things," I wondered, "How could I set matters right for them?" I'd come to Central America, like so many others, out of a vague sense of compassion, a desire to be of service. There's a hard American edge to all that: an unshakeable confidence in technique, a dogmatic faith that things can be controlled, fixed. The gringo takes apart whatever seems to be the problem, sees how it works, then puts it back together the right way. That, at least, is the plan.

Scott Cairns has a poem called "Late Results," which explores the world we've made with all our well-intentioned tinkering. In the poem, the halt and lame get hip replacements, the hungry grow fat (while remaining hungry), and orphans learn to fend for themselves. The few remaining prophets think themselves mad and keep silent. The poem ends: "Only the poor—who are with us always—only they continued in the hope."[1]

I try to put my finger on the meaning of that phrase, "continued in the hope," but it slips away to lurk in shadows of poetic opacity. This I know: there's a difference between hope and optimism, that sunny North American certainty that ingenuity and grit will, as sure as day follows night, make things better. Hope longs and works confidently for the better, but claims no certainty save that days come and go. The most hopeful people I've met have no reason to cling to fantasies of progress, and hold close to each other and the place they know as home. The hopeful know whom they belong to, even when alone. They know where they come from, even in a strange land.

As a doctor, I wanted to offer something more concrete than hope. At the very least, I like to know what I'm up against. The first, anxious hour with Jenrry in the treatment room was a welcome change from the riddles of caring for Roberto. With Jenrry—at least at first—I knew where we were: my patient was in shock. I knew what we had to do to keep him from dying. We congratulated ourselves for snatching him from death with our science and technology. But then he crossed into another story, a country where the terrain was strange, unstable, threatening to explode with volcanic fury. No longer at ease with promises of control, we fell back on hope, where the poor have always lived.

Roberto was one of the poorest people I've met. I've told his story many times now. Most listeners say little. Recounting personal encounters with starving children isn't a great conversation starter. When I get a response, it's often to propose a big solution: economic reforms, social justice,

---

1. Cairns, "Late Results," in *Slow Pilgrim: The Collected Poems,* 166.

changes "those people" must carry out with guidance and a little help from the North. All of these would be very helpful, I'm sure, and cost me very little. Great minds have been working on them for years. On rare occasions, someone suggests changes in US government policy, though not in the behavior of its citizens. I've yet to hear anyone ask, "What do Hondurans say should be done?"

Limiting our responses to technological or policy fixes to help "those people" dodges hard questions: How much comfort and control are people living in developed countries prepared to give up so those who live in hope can get simply get by? Does my passion for justice fall off precisely when it starts to cost me something? Questions like these keep Jenrry and Roberto with me. Hope, after all, is more costly than it is comforting. When I remember the dark abyss of Roberto's gaze or Jennry's wan smile, I feel a fierce, demanding hope. It's what I find in many Honduran souls, nothing at all like cheery optimism. It's a hope the screwed and shafted of the world know, a birthright, a staple crop suited to harsh soil.

The time came at last for me to return to my own country. Leaving Antigua for Guatemala City, I rode the tourist shuttle and stared from my cushioned seat at ramshackle "chicken buses" jammed with passengers in the pre-dawn darkness. We arrived at the airport on time, everything in order. I checked in, paid the exit fees, and walked to the gate. There was time to kill. I bought a cooked breakfast, a cup of good coffee. I sat down to read a book.

The most difficult moment in any of my trips south is the return. There are helpful absurdities along the way, of course: expensive cars on display in a Honduran airport or shelves of duty-free luxuries for sale in a country where children starve. I've learned to take it in slowly, like a diver rising in stages from the ocean, pausing at set depths to avoid the bends. Even so, returning leaves me dizzy, disoriented, lost. Grim-faced travelers race to catch their flights, grumble at perceived inconveniences, absent-mindedly thumb retail goods and souvenirs along the concourse, toss half-eaten meals in the trash. "Please," I say to myself, "don't let me be like those people," knowing all along I'm one of them. In two weeks, I'll be fully re-absorbed. I'll walk grocery store aisles, confident the world truly needs ten brands of underarm deodorant and three varieties of diet cat food. I'll grab something to eat—fried, fatty, and fast—and swallow it quickly, not stopping to think of the land that grew what I've eaten or the hands through which my food passed. I might even forget all I've seen and heard were it not for people I've come to know along the way. I knew them only briefly, but can't shake them. Thank God for that. When I feel completely at ease in the controlled artificiality of the place I call home, they haunt me once again. They bless me with fierce hope.

Chapter Thirteen

Wendell and Me

*Cincinnati, Ohio/Departamento
de Intibucá, Honduras*

IN THAT LITERATURE AND medicine elective I taught, fourth year medical students read fiction, memoirs, essays and plays about health, disease, physicians and patients. Our goal was to connect these works with the lives of the doctors in training. Most attempts were encouraging; some less so. From the beginning, we read works by the Kentucky farmer, writer, and conservationist, Wendell Berry. They were not well received.

One student dismissed Berry's essay, "Health is Membership," as "most revolting thing I've ever been forced to read." Others were troubled with Berry's attention to—as they saw it—trivial details of hospital experience: poor food and bad sleeping conditions. The strongest objections, though, focused on Berry's criticism that medicine, in emphasizing technological solutions derived from fallible and often misapplied science, destroys human connections between patients, communities, and the land. "Who does this Kentucky farmer think he is, telling me how to be a doctor?" complained one. To Berry's claim that "medicine is an exact science until applied,"[1] another countered: "Medicine *is* an exact science, and it's getting more exact all the time," as if that negated Berry's troubling word, "until . . ." A second-generation immigrant went further, pounding her fist on the table as she declared, "The reason American medicine's the best in world is

1. Berry, "Health is Membership," in *Another Turn of the Crank,* 106.

158

capitalism!" She didn't elaborate, nor did I ask by what criteria she assessed America's medical superiority, though I might have called to her attention many public health measures, such as infant mortality, teen pregnancy, and health care access, in which the United States' world ranking is shameful.

Still, I was grateful our students responded to the text, if not necessarily as I would have liked. Their reactions persuaded me that challenging ideas are more readily received as story than direct statement. While some complained about medically "unrealistic" descriptions in Berry's short story, "Fidelity," in which family members rescue the dying Burley Coulter from a Louisville hospital so he may die with his own people in his own country, the fictional narrative spurred less protest than the essay. They neutralized even the story's critique, though, telling me that improved doctor-patient communication and the end of what they've been trained to call paternalism made "Fidelity" a relic of a best-forgotten past. I wondered if they work in the same hospitals as I do. It was clear, however, that students about to begin the long, often grueling, years of residency training were poorly disposed toward criticism of the profession, even if medical practice has precious little to profess these days.

Some students liked Berry's work. One recalled his own days on a Kentucky farm and how he relished walking the woods in peace after a frenetic week in the hospital. I even found residents reading Berry on their own, though they tend to be an odd sort in this business. After all, they were reading something other than online medical references and journal articles, and a resident's schedule rarely permits leisure reading. Some came from small towns or farms. They found Berry attractive because he offered an alternative voice to that of the mainstream medical industry. Not that they bought all of Berry's critique. One young doctor I met on a medical trip to Honduras said, "Yeah, I really like what he has to say, except that story about stealing the guy from the hospital. That was just wild."

Is Wendell Berry too wild for medicine? My corner of the medical profession betrays little awareness of an organic link between community and health. Families visiting my office come from an array of economic and ethnic backgrounds. Most of my patients can't afford private medical insurance. Some drive many miles and wait in a lobby full of strangers before being seen. At best, my patients and I weave in and out of each other's lives. Our interactions are vignettes in parallel but unrelated dramas.

On a busy afternoon, for example, after saying goodbye to a mother whose healthy newborn has just made his first visit, I walk down the hall and grab the next chart: a fifteen-year-old male, here for a sports physical. Entering, I find he's alone. He stares at me from his seat atop the exam table, arms crossed, looking annoyed. He's more wiry than muscular, with a heavy dose of mistrust and insecurity in his stony glare. I take a seat; start asking questions. His answers are telegraphically brief: no problems, school's boring, basketball this winter. To keep in playing form, he avoids tobacco, but likes marijuana, preferring it to alcohol. We talk about this. I give him the facts as I know them, along with advice I doubt he'll take. He's learned much from the economy, from movies, television, and music. I ask him to talk with his parents, but he says his mother has her own troubles and he hasn't seen his father in months. Teachers and counselors can't be trusted. He's experienced and makes his own decisions.

I ask, "When's the last time you had sex?" He glares and spits out a line he's been rehearsing since his arrival, "I was supposed to get some this afternoon, and you're keeping me from it." He's showing off, though I don't doubt he's seen far more than I did at his age. My job, according to the experts, is to suggest other ways of behaving—though he has little incentive to change— and offer him technologies to reduce the harm he causes himself and others. We talk "safe sex," "protection," and birth control. It's old news to him. He knows how to get condoms, shows no interest in contraception. I don't mention how rarely a teen mother in my practice seeks child support from the baby's father. I ask instead what he wants from life, which turns out to be an NBA career, lots of consumer electronics, and endless autonomy. His eyes tell me I'm pressing too hard. I'm here as his pediatric specialist, period. He wants what he came for. At the end of the visit, I sign his sports form—he is, after all, physically able to play—and urge him to make an appointment so we can discuss these things again. If he returns, I'll be shocked.

I step in to the hallway, where the office social worker has been waiting for me. The functionally illiterate mother I referred to her last month missed another appointment. The social worker asks how hard to press in locating her, reminding me we don't have a working telephone number for this family. We both know Child Protective Services is stretched too thin to pursue cases without evidence of abuse or serious medical neglect. This family simply needs help, and I don't know where to get it for them. Now I don't even know where in this medium-sized city to find the family.

I return to the doctor's charting room, where a colleague mentions another of my patients, a sixteen-year-old girl named Crys, whom he saw in follow-up yesterday, when I was out of the office. I've never met Crys's father. Her grandmother used to bring her in when she was younger, but Crys resented her grandmother's "nosiness." Now she comes alone. If it's serious, she brings her mother. I've spent time with Crys, investigating her many physical complaints and reinforcing the importance of good choices, a consumer phrase she's comfortable with. Sex holds little mystery for her.

Sex is something the men in her life apparently expect from her, though she offers no hint of enjoying it, so we focus on "protection" and birth control. We've talked over a number of methods, and she's tried several, with lots of encouragement and scheduled follow-up visits. There's no knowledge deficit with Crys. She knows more about contraception in her mid-teens than I did entering medical school. The news from my colleague is that he's made an appointment for her with the teen pregnancy clinic. She might keep this baby. Of course, that's what Crys told me a year ago, before her first abortion. I remember taking a long time then with her and her mother, asking about community supports—extended family, friends, adoption agencies, church. They listened to what I said, then told me none of these fit their needs.

If I seem to focus on sexual behavior, it's part of the job description for anyone who cares for adolescents. I'm not so naïve to imagine teen sexual abstinence as an historical norm. Long before the Montagues and Capulets just said no, long before the word *adolescent* was invented, and long, long before this particular consumer demographic was scientifically mapped for maximal corporate exploitation, teenagers have been, to use the fashionable term, sexually active. What troubles me is the way the experience of sex is now shaped by consumer expectations—one more technologically modified private activity divorced from sustained concern for people or place.

Nor is sex the only part of life lately reshaped to the contours of consumer control and choice. When I ask young children where their food comes from, few can tell me what precedes the grocery store. Most of my patients know more about singers and sports stars than about their next-door neighbors. Mothers kiss their children on the steps of the day care center, hoping they'll be well looked after while Mommy's at school or work. Fathers—at least those actually involved in their children's lives—are similarly caught in a brutal economy of getting and spending. But when, amid this frantic using up of manufactured products and contrived experiences, do children learn to ponder the mystery of their own lives or cultivate affection for the nonfungible things of this world? Where—outside of movies, television, and popular songs—does anyone learn to love?

It seems love, like sex, is thought to come naturally, as if a practice so complex demanded less than a people's sustained effort. Like any worthwhile human practice—health or peace, for example—love is hard work. To thrive, it needs more than a chance. It was Father Zosima, the ascetic monk in Dostoevsky's *Brothers Karamazov* who said, "Love in action is a harsh and dreadful thing compared with love in dreams."[2] I'm not sure how

2. Dostoevsky, *The Brothers Karamazov*, 55.

many of my patients—or my own children, for that matter—would turn to a monk, if they knew where to find one, for advice on love. That even one of them would seriously entertain the possibility of living like monks—side by side, in community, and for life—is probably beyond imagining.

My patients generally buy the aggressively marketed American dogma of individual autonomy. So do their parents, who see autonomy as central to health, with the corresponding fear that incapacity and age turn each of us into "a burden." That we might already burden the world with heedless consumption or burden our neighbors with unlimited material demands is left unexplored. An endless craving for autonomy leaves my patients disconnected from one another and defenseless against the scientifically calibrated power of marketers. The unstated price of our autonomy is estranging solitude, a loneliness hidden even from ourselves with the help of electronic diversions and chemical comforts.

These are the concerns that stay with me when I leave the office. They're what I bring to the page when I read Wendell Berry. I share his doubt that a place can start with isolated, autonomous individuals and arrive at wholeness. I sit up and pay attention when he writes in an aphoristic essay on—of all things—the specialization of poetry, that to be autonomous "is to be 'broken off and separate.'"[3] For Berry, the state of our literature is connected to the state of our land, our economy, our neighborhoods, and our health. In an age of specialization, professional turf wars and fortified intellectual fiefdoms, Berry is a marauding generalist.

I'm a pediatrician. I specialize in the medical care of children. I considered a host of pediatric subgenres before accepting I was and remain a generalist among "baby doctors." My students are well on their way to specializing, choosing fields within which many will later subspecialize. It makes sense within the complex medical system to narrow one's focus and master the powerful tools of a single, well-defined discipline. The best subspecialists remain keenly interested in general care, but professional, intellectual, and economic pressures drive nearly all to limit their practice. The effect on the imagination is rather like the story of the elephant and the blind men, each of whom understood the elephant to be that part of the animal they had touched and, in a fashion, comprehended: the tusk, the trunk, the flank, the tail. It's a funny story, but only to those who already know what an elephant looks like, alive and whole. As the medical joke goes, a nephrologist sees the heart as a pump supplying the kidneys with blood. Having dismembered the body its component systems, it's but a simple step to envision the body as a machine assembled from smaller, systemic

3. Berry, "Notes: Unspecializing Poetry," in *Standing by Words*, 80.

modules. The whole is lost in its component parts. In this view, the heart is not only like a pump; it is one. It can even be replaced by a machine pump, though not for long and only at an astonishing cost. Likewise, kidneys are conceptually transformed into enormously complex filters, the eye, a camera, and the brain a meat computer. Yet, as the Kentucky farmer reminds the body's technicians, the machine analogy, like all analogies, ultimately fails: "Divided from its sources of air, food, drink, clothing, shelter and companionship, a body is, properly speaking, a cadaver, whereas a machine by itself, shut down or out of fuel, is still a machine."[4]

The paradox of specialized medicine, then, is that I gain enormous power from understanding the complexities of the body in isolation, while the embodied, social organism withers as communal context is stripped away. My patients are measured, medicated and—in a fashion—nourished in isolation from the land that produces our food. Not surprisingly, isolation and misplaced confidence in technology disturb all human experience, including language. Specialized technique requires useful vocabulary: words that produce desired effects. Doctors are, after all, highly trained professionals. But what my patients and their parents often want, in addition to expertise, is useable information in understandable language in order to make informed decisions about care. I listen as residents translate highly specialized information into layman's terms—how vocabulary reveals our pretensions!—while words spanning entire continents of human experience are banished from the medical encounter: love, friendship, mercy. Clumsy attempts to graft words like *intimacy* onto a conversation about "safe sex" are soon revealed as halfhearted afterthoughts. Intimacy, like love or friendship, can be a starting place, a journey, and a destination—words rendered meaningless without a particular place in the created world to stand on— but it's none of these things when spliced into a purely instrumental activity. As for *mercy*, I've heard the word used in a medical context but once: in that appalling oxymoron, "mercy killing," an obsolete term for what's now called physician-assisted suicide.

Unlike the medical students, I came to Berry's work after several years in the profession, already mystified by medicine's absurdities. If I, like them, had read his work as a student, I might have rejected it as an ill-informed diatribe. Had I read it in the gloomy depths of residency, I might have used it as a means to blame medicine for my personal unhappiness. I might even have left medicine entirely to search out some rural utopia that would have, in the end, left me just as unhappy. I was fortunate to discover Berry's

4. Berry, "Health is Membership," in *Another Turn of the Crank,* 94–95.

writing when I could read it critically. Berry made explicit what I, at best, half-understood: that mischief follows whenever technology-dependent, specialized medicine separates bodies from community. Of course, Berry isn't unique in finding things amiss in modern medicine, though others often misdiagnose the problem. The contemporary emphasis on individualized health assumes that patient isolation is a side effect best treated homeopathically, using increments of the existing malady. The wounds created by illusions of autonomy are patched over with new choices for the autonomous consumer: concierge medical practices, doctor-approved complementary medicine, and birthing rooms remodeled to resemble suburban boudoirs.

This banquet of choice is typically available only to a fortunate few living in technology-rich northern countries. The way in which specialized, technology-dependent medicine obscures and destroys embodied connection is clearer in the so-called developing world. There's an implicit assumption in our terminology that "developed" is superior to "developing." That may be true in some respects. I'm pleased my doctor has all the medicine and equipment she needs to care for me. I must avoid unnecessarily privileging the primitive. But the implied trajectory of what's called "development" assumes northern countries are models, goals toward which the rest of the world should aim. At the same time, such terminology hides the real costs of technology and development on the lives of those not directly benefiting from them.

When I'm in Honduras, I'm simply a doctor, not a specialist. I provide medical care for all comers. On one medical trip to Honduras, I saw patients while another university team began the complex task of establishing a new clinic in a mountain village. The clinic had a wood stove and a few electric lights, but no running water. We joined the villagers in line to use the town pump, stewarding every drop for our drinking, cooking, and bathing. Yet to the side the town square was, of all things, an Internet café. After long hours treating intestinal parasites, bandaging machete wounds, or delivering babies by flashlight, we paid a few lempiras and left behind the distressing confines of material reality. Perhaps the Internet had delivered on its promise: we were instantly in touch with the world. Yet that was and has always been a con, an illusion. For all the excitement of emailing loved ones, there was, in fact, no one to touch, nothing present to us save a plastic box, a glowing screen.

Late one afternoon, a group of us visited a *pulperia* and bought chocobananas: frozen chocolate-covered fruit on a stick. Kevin, one of the residents, struck up a conversation outside the shop with a woman holding a thin-looking infant. He learned the baby was the woman's nephew, whose mother had died soon after the child's birth. The father, we were told, was unreliable and rarely around, so the baby's aunt took the infant in. She had no money for formula and lived several hours' walk from town. They were very poor. Reliable food and water were hard to come by. Kevin borrowed my equipment and examined the baby. He had an ear infection, was mildly dehydrated, and almost certainly had parasites stealing what calories he swallowed. Our makeshift pharmacy was just up the hill, from which we gathered medicines and rehydrating solution for the baby to drink. We had very little baby formula, but could get more from our main clinic two hour's drive away. Kevin explained all this to the grateful woman, now softly crying as she held the baby to her chest. He arranged for her to come by the government health center the next day, where he would re-examine the child and give them more formula. We would introduce her then to the local health workers, who could explore other ways to support her. We stayed to talk with her awhile, then headed back up the hill, feeling less self-congratulatory that we'd done a good deed than worried we hadn't done nearly enough.

Most of the human needs we encounter are beyond a doctor's power to satisfy. The lasting solution to diarrhea and parasites isn't medicine, but readily available clean water. Chronic malnutrition won't be eliminated with IVs and high-dose multivitamins, but with reliable and affordable food. Crushing poverty demands new ways to make a living that don't cripple bodies or wound the land. I have no medicine for such things. No individual does. A certain amount of technology will help, to be sure, but what's obvious to me when in rural Honduras is that community trumps technology.

That same evening, I joined Sarah, one of the nurses, on the tiled landing of the municipal building our group was using as the women's dormitory. We sipped Honduran coffee and talked over the day's events, looking down on the town square and up to the rugged hills surrounding us. Even in dry season, the slopes were green and lush in the evening light. I remembered the perceptual trick I'd learned on my first Honduran expedition: things look beautiful at a distance; it's only close up that you see the suffering. Sarah pointed out the trash littering the town square: plastic bags, boxes, popsicle sticks, and paper scattered like treats for an Easter egg hunt. The few trashcans—prominently labeled with slogans about keeping the village healthy and beautiful—overflowed. Sarah asked what it would take to instill enough pride in the townspeople for them care about appearances. I wondered, in response, if the litter didn't cast judgment as much on American culture—throwaway items being visible markers of our economy—that increasing access to electronic media encouraged the locals to emulate. In my experience, Hondurans aren't necessarily inclined to conserve when readily available consumer products make careful husbandry unnecessary.

Given the choice, they throw away plastic wrapping as thoughtlessly as their wealthy neighbors to the north. Compared to North Americans, however, they're less likely to forget the earth's material limits, if only because they lack the wealth and mobility to do so for long. Necessity and scarcity make demanding tutors.

At the end of the brigade, on the bus ride north to the airport, we passed banana plantations and vast fields from which sugar cane had been harvested. The first time I saw this fertile valley—six years earlier—was shortly after the catastrophic floods accompanying Hurricane Mitch. Then, the corporately owned fields lay barren, while displaced locals occupied shantytowns snaking along the highway median from San Pedro Sula—the business and HIV capital of Honduras—to El Progreso, a city of uncommon squalor.

This time, though, the plantations were flourishing, while the once displaced locals had reassumed their accustomed invisibility. With a copy of Berry's *Citizenship Papers* in hand, I was in the mood to raise irksome questions. Which, I wondered, was stranger: a village with no running water sporting an Internet café, or entire valleys devoted to large scale export monoculture in a country struggling to feed its own people? Some Hondurans living in the valley were, no doubt, employed by multinational corporations supplying the wealthy North with inexpensive fruit and sugar. Doubtless, too, Honduran government officials and private citizens profited from this arrangement. Still, I had difficulty understanding why the underfed children I treated the day before couldn't benefit from the land's agricultural abundance. Perhaps the world economy is best served using this rich bottomland as one exploitable resource among others around the globe. I lack the macroeconomic language and training to refute such assertions. This much, though, was quite clear: one part of the world suffered harm for the benefit of another, which happened to be mine.

The smell of burning sugar cane hung in the air as we stepped off the bus at the airport. It had rained more than anticipated in the dry season and the cane fields were being torched later than usual. The result was a brown particulate haze throughout the valley, dense enough to ground commercial jet traffic. The plane we were supposed to board for our flight home never landed in San Pedro Sula. After an initial approach, it was redirected north to the States. As trip leaders scrambled for alternatives, others asked what was going on. When I explained about the burning cane fields, one of our crew said, knowingly, "So we're trapped here because of their economy." A voice, sounding rather like a Kentucky farmer, spoke sharply in my head: "No, we're trapped because of *our* economy." No matter what my colleague and I had done for the people of Honduras, we were sugar consumers, and the land serving as a sugar factory had to be readied for next year's production. Had we remained in the States, the consequences of our consumptive habits, now causing us momentary inconvenience, would have remained invisible. That these same habits might trap others in permanent misery was more than any of us wanted to know.

In such times, a technologically-dependent man like me—raised to believe that specialized knowledge, properly applied, will shape any reality to human desire—hopes the world's connections and limits can be either be transcended or ignored. Trained over many years to consume the things of this world with no thought to their provenance, I join my fellow North Americans in pillaging our planet and bodies. No affection for created things is required to bend nature to our will and ignore the damage done in the process. When I work on the Navajo reservation or in Honduras, I'm physically present to the damage done. I read it with my eyes. I listen with my ears.

I use my body and senses to diagnose, treat, and reassure. Placing the diaphragm of my stethoscope on the chest of the febrile child, I listen for the rustle of breath, the murmur of a heart. I touch the pads of my fingers to a frightened adolescent's wrist, taking her pulse. I watch amazed at the ferocity with which a hungry infant nurses at his mother's breast. I stir with passions that, despite Dr. Osler's warning, ground my compassion. I am an embodied creature working among other such creatures. It took years to learn that only by nurturing affection for these others can I rightly serve them, much less understand what it means to be healthy. It may take more than a lifetime to unlearn the dogmas of a consumptive economy. I struggle –usually without effect—to see the world through the eyes of Francis of Assisi, who knew every creature, animate and inanimate, as brother or sister. Siblings in a healthy community don't ask reasons why they should care for one another, nor do they permit anyone to abuse family members.

We do well to acknowledge such relationships, make them explicit rather than obscure. Technology's power to mask relationships is, perhaps, its least appreciated attribute. I'm a better doctor when I work on the Navajo Reservation, and a better doctor in rural Central America than when I'm in a US city. I can be better present to my patients in places where I'm stripped of the trappings of the medical-industrial complex, where we face each other on something resembling an equal footing. It is important to admit, though, that such nakedness reduces my effectiveness, at least in terms North Americans have been taught to measure effectiveness: convenience, longevity, and material comfort.

It's natural for me to desire these things. I want my patients to live, and technology helps that happen. I hope, however, that my patients teach me to complain less when my own desires are frustrated. Saint Augustine, who knew something of frustrated desire, was drawn to the Manichaean religion—which divided the universe into blessed spirit and gross matter—because he believed, for a time, that it best explained the gulf between the world he desired and the world in which he lived. The Manichaean subordination of matter to spirit—not too different, perhaps, than believing pure reason will eliminate human misery—promised a way past earthly limits. Yet, in Book VII of *Confessions*, Augustine records his late discovery of the created world's goodness. For him, the evil that mars creation names, not a presence, but an absence, a deprivation of the good. From this moment on, he took all creation seriously, no longer dividing the desired from the undesired: "I no longer wished for a better world, because I was thinking of the *whole* of creation."[5]

Augustine, keenly aware of the *Ordo Amoris*, the right-ordering of loves, struggled to order his many earthly loves. For Augustine, everything—including the professions—properly honors and serves higher things. Taking Augustine's cue, Wendell Berry has Wheeler Catlett, the small town lawyer in "Fidelity," advise the confused Detective Bode on the proper use of the law:

> "But, my dear boy, you don't eat or drink the law, or sit in the
> shade of it or warm yourself by it, or wear it, or have your being
> in it. The law exists only to serve."
> "Serve what?"
> "Why, all the things that are above it. Love."[6]

Wheeler Catlett knows something Detective Bode does not: things are never as discrete and separable as we wish, that autonomy and specialization, for all their productive power, cause mischief and harm apart from an embodied affection for a contextual whole. We learn to care for those things we attend to directly and over time, the intricate web of creatures that affect us and for which we, in turn, grow in affection. Wheeler, who chides Bode after the detective angrily accuses Danny Branch of burying Burley, "somewhere in these end-of-nowhere, godforsaken hills and hollows,"[7] also knows something about finding grace and holiness even in the end-of-nowhere places of the created world.

Yet, like a broken clock, Detective Bode couldn't help but be right on occasion. Danny did, in fact, bury Burley Coulter in the hills the old man

---

5. St. Augustine, *Confessions*, Book VII, Chapter 13, my own, somewhat free, translation, emphasis added.

6. Wendell Berry, "Fidelity," in *That Distant Land*, 418.

7. Ibid., 427.

loved. Danny, who understands the landscape as anything but "godforsaken," returns after the burial to a Port William membership with "the aspect and the brightness of one who had borne the dead to the grave, and filled the grave to the brim, and received the dead back into life again."[8]

"Receiving the dead back into life again," seems rather much for the American medical system to take on right now. Perhaps, though, there is something to be learned from a community reclaiming one of its members from an overconfident medical industry. That's what my patients do for me.

When in Honduras, I particularly enjoy working with our interpreters, Honduran students from a privileged, English-speaking school who give up their vacation time to help us. One of them, a loud and funny young woman who liked to dance and tell jokes, was a particular favorite of mine on one trip. She was not conventionally beautiful. She was too fond, I suppose, of good food to become another surgically-enhanced fashion wraith. But no one could deny she was beautiful, her body overflowing with life, her face betraying true delight in nearly everything she saw. She and I often told stories outside the clinic after the last patient had been seen. We laughed nearly as often as we spoke. On our last day in the village, as we gathered our belongings for the trip home, she handed me a postcard, signed by all the interpreters but written in her own hand, which read in part, "Thank you for loving my country and my people."

Love is a word doctors rarely use. It's not in Osler's canon of medical virtues. I thought back to my first visit to Honduras after Hurricane Mitch and the people I met who left me so uncomfortable, no longer at ease in my old life. I thought of the many children I'd met here, the little I'd done to help them, the links they unknowingly forged between their lives and mine. I remembered sawtoothed horizons in the Honduran mountains, the scent of burning cane, the taste of mango fresh from the tree, the voices of welcome and hospitality I'd done nothing to deserve.

I had a fondness for all of this, but did I really love them? Was *love* the right word? I've worked in Honduras, in a particular place and with particular people, long and often enough to hazard an answer. I love her country. I love her people.

Which brings us to a starting place.

8. Ibid., 426.

Chapter Fourteen

Silence

Abiquiu, New Mexico/
Cincinnati, Ohio

AT FIVE THIRTY A.M. I step from the warmth of my room onto the narrow covered porch. I reach back inside to turn off the light, and close the door behind me. I'm not yet fully awake, and a yawn ends in unexpected shivers. The desert air is bracingly cold. A single lamp glows in a far room of the guesthouse. The not-quite-Passover moon has already sunk below the canyon wall. I pause for my eyes to adjust to the meager available light, then set foot on the gravelly courtyard to take in my ghostly surroundings. Degrees of darkness define the land. My eyes turn to the cloudless night sky, where the constellation Scorpius curls above the southeastern horizon. Its brightest star, the red supergiant Antares, glimmers at the scorpion's heart near sweeping diagonals of the Milky Way. The light from Antares traveled 550 years to reach my eye. I'm seeing the past: photons hurled earth's way before Columbus thought of sailing west to the Indies, before Motecuhzoma II ruled the Aztec Empire, and before Martin Luther donned the robes of an Augustinian friar. The hazy light of the Milky Way is far older, having crossed silent vacancies too vast for me to comprehend. To the west, a twenty-first century satellite moves in a stately arc between canyon walls, reflecting light from the unseen Sun. A single meteor flames earthward in self-erasure. I breathe in the silence of infinite spaces. I'm unafraid but trembling, and it's not clear whether from the cold or out of joy, standing in so vast a mystery.

The sky is lovely, dark, and deep, but I haven't risen early to stargaze. I'm walking uphill, toward the chapel of the Monastery of Christ in the Desert, barely distinguishable from the shadowy canyon wall behind by a soft light from its clerestory windows. I'm on my way to chapel for Lauds, second of the canonical hours—set times when monks gather to pray. Benedictines pray together seven times daily and fill the day's remainder with manual labor, meals taken in silence, quiet contemplation, and *lectio divina*. The monks have been up for hours. I've already missed Vigils, having slept through the 3:40 a.m. bell. I'm too fond of sleep to be a good monk.

Shivering under spring stars, I climb the dirt road toward the chapel. I've forgotten a flashlight, so I step lightly to avoid rocks, potholes, and cow pies on the way. I pull the zipper of my fleece to the top of the upturned collar and bury my hands in my pockets. Every ten paces or so, I stop, crane my neck, and receive this place.

If river level in Grand Canyon is my favorite spot in the universe, this wide bank of the Rio Chama in New Mexico is a close second. The river is to my left, unseen in the darkness, bearing its red-ochre cargo of mud toward the Rio Grande. A small cemetery is ahead. Upstream lie vegetable gardens and enclosed fields where the monks grow hops and lavender: products they sell to support their life. Much thought and effort goes toward sustainable use of limited resources: straw bale construction, passive solar design, photovoltaic panels, solar heating, and creative water conservation. When needs exceed income, they go without.

The monks make a vow of stability to this community in a place of ample sun and scarce water. They find and make beauty in simple things. Any extravagances here are found in lavish Benedictine hospitality toward guests and the adobe chapel designed by the late architect and woodworker, George Nakashima. At first glance, the chapel looks simple: a bell tower, adobe walls, thirty-foot high clerestory panels in four directions. Thomas Merton, the Trappist monk, poet, and author who stopped here on his 1968 trip to Asia, marveled at how elegantly Nakashima fit his lines and surfaces into the surrounding cliffs, making for interest from all angles and times of day.

In the predawn darkness, I see the chapel only as light from the upper windows and looming shadow below, but as I climb the steps to the front entrance, a motion-activated lamp snaps on, illuminating the unadorned portico. I stamp dirt from my shoes before pulling the wooden door open to enter the lit chapel interior. Two fellow retreatants sit in the rows of wooden chairs by the entrance. A few monks are already in the choir stalls on either side of the altar. I bow toward the altarpiece, take my seat, and pick up a choir book, opening it to this morning's Lauds.

From behind the free-standing sanctuary altarpiece, draped in purple
for the season of Lent, monks silently emerge, one by one or in small groups,
bowing before taking their places in the choir stalls. They range in age from
barely twenty to more than eighty and come from North and South America,
Europe, Africa, South and East Asia. In all-black habits, they look like flock-
ing ravens and prove just as difficult to tell one from another at first. In time,
though, one learns their distinctive marks and behaviors, much the way one
identifies wild birds. Years of communal prayer, work, contemplation, and
obedience paradoxically render each monk more singular than most of us
on the outside, obsessively preening our individualism and autonomy.

I whisper the names of the monks as they enter: Brother Bernard,
Brother Jude, Brother Francis, Brother Andre, Brother Christian, the two
Brothers Benedict. Others arrive whom I know by sight but not by name.
Last comes Abbot Philip with his gap-toothed smile. He finds his place on
the left choir stall, taps the wooden frame, and we rise in unison to sing.

I've come here for a few days of silence and contemplative prayer. Not
a polite sip, but a hard pull: straight with no chaser, what the late Walter
Burghardt called, "a long loving look at the real."[1] The monastery is an obser-
vatory where the telescopes are the eye, ear, mind, and heart. I've just completed a month's work on the Navajo Reservation, seeing patients in Tuba
City and supervising pediatric residents in Gallup, New Mexico. What could
have been nothing more than a *locum tenens* job was instead a re-immersion
in a place and its people: the soft speech of Navajo children, the smell of fry
bread and mutton, the long horizontals of waterless plateaus. It feels increasingly like home again, though a month away from Jill grows tiresome and
lonely. I want to go to her, but before I do, I pause for a few days to empty
myself in the rhythms of this place and dwell with others in silence.

The monks come for a lifetime, seeking a life of prayer, work, and
stability. They come to find truth and lose themselves. They come to live
vowed lives of obedience (from the Latin, *oboedire*, "to listen attentively, give
ear,") and community (from *communis*, "common, shared"). Some eventually leave for other communities. Others discover that their calling here was
a mistake or one stop in a long journey, and return to their previous lives.
Many will stay to join their predecessors buried in the cemetery near the
chapel.

When I ask monks why they entered this vocation, they speak of great
need and profound longing. Not one tells me they came because they felt
spiritually advanced, unusually gifted, or particularly holy. Wise monks

1. Burghardt, "Contemplation: A Long Loving Look at the Real," in ed. Traub, *An
Ignatian Spirituality Reader,* 89.

learn to laugh at themselves. They know they'll often fail. That's why they live together. When one stumbles, the others—often the ones they find most annoying—help them back to their feet. Everything a monk hopes to leave behind in the world comes with him. If they meant to flee their personal failings, they're soon disillusioned. If they sought an easy life, free from distractions, they chose poorly. A monk once told me his second greatest obstacle to a holy life was other monks: "You have no idea how unbearable someone's loud chewing becomes after fifteen years eating at the same table."

The greatest obstacle, he said, was himself.

The monk devotes a lifetime to three mysteries he has no hope of understanding: God, neighbor, and self. In time, even the self—at least that part the psychologically-inclined might call "ego"—becomes as much an Other as the rest. When Tony O'Brien, a photojournalist, lived and prayed with monks at Christ in the Desert while documenting their lives in pictures, he wondered what kept these men here when so many other choices seemed more attractive. One monk told him how disconcerting it was to realize, two weeks into his stay, that he'd be sharing this space with the same people for the rest of his life. Abbot Philip said, "In a monastery like this, you have to grow or you have to leave, because we don't have any outlets. A contemplative community simply focuses on the interior life, period. One must take a real personal approach. It's like a marriage or any relationship."[2]

In addition to hours of prayer, that focus "on the interior life, period," happens through (not in spite of) living, working, and eating together—again, like a marriage. The Navajo may get it right in naming marriage, "getting used to each other." I've heard *bilagáanas* protest that there's no romance in a term that doesn't mention love, but where might love be learned—much less sustained—except in the hard, everyday work of living out shared commitments and practices? I'm a lifelong Beatles fan, but to imagine all I need is love is as naïve as thinking peace needs nothing more than a chance. Love—like peace or the profession of medicine—is hard work, sustained in gritty and unsentimental practices that shape the persons who embody them. Monks come to the community aware they are possessed of habits too corrupt for the love their shared life demands. They come as much to unlearn old habits as to embrace new ones. They begin to love those they once considered unlovable. They learn firsthand the truth spoken by Dostoevsky's Father Zosima: "Love in action is a harsh and dreadful thing compared with love in dreams."[3] Monks live and grow into love through encounters with the

2. O'Brien, *Light in the Desert*, 30.
3. Dosteovsky, *The Brothers Karamazov*, 55.

ultimately unknowable Others they share their lives with. Whatever else a monastery may be, it's a school of difficult love.

* * * *

I tell pediatric residents and medical students on rounds, "You have to love your patients, even those you can't bring yourself to like." I should say it more often, but it has a disorienting effect on professionals not used to hearing the word "love" in the same conversation as "non-gap metabolic acidosis" or "late infantile metachromatic leukodystrophy." Doctors are, after all, champions of instrumental reason, and my profession's well-policed boundaries exile so-called subjective matters like love to the private realm. I try to convey to the residents my own hard-earned lessons: that genuine affection turns abstract patients into persons and that love is necessary, though insufficient, to good doctoring. Necessary because my patients require and deserve affection, even at their worst. Insufficient because they require competent medical care.

When I tell residents, "love your patients," I have no idea how they take it. When I was their age, the word "love" careened between the pornographic and sentimental, twin poles I mistook for opposites. To the degree abstract love summoned images of the body, they focused on highly idealized and very specific parts. Today, however, when I say the words "patient" and "love" in the same sentence, I see very specific persons and entire, if not necessarily complete, bodies. Sometimes I see Khalil, Roberto, or Jenrry. Other times, I see Jasmine and wonder if I've learned anything about love.

Jasmine came to my office in a custom wheelchair, fitted with head supports, padding to keep her back straight and prevent pressure ulcers, and a rabbit's warren of bins in which her mother stored necessities for their excursions. Though Jasmine was old enough for junior high, she rarely attended her "severe-to-profound" special education class in the public school because she was so susceptible to viral illnesses acquired from her classmates. A simple cold might worsen her seizures or progress to pneumonia, landing her in the hospital for days.

Her objective intellectual abilities were those of an infant or toddler, the result of what her medical history called "cerebral palsy." A look at a CT of her head, however, was frightening. I'm familiar enough with brain images to search them for familiar structures the way one seeks recognizable coastlines and borders on a map. When the expected contours aren't there, I look for distortions, missing pieces, or other signs of disease. But Jasmine's CT wasn't merely distorted. There was a black emptiness where normal brain ought to be and a thin white rim of cerebral cortex just beneath the skull, looking less like a jumbled map than the gaseous remnant of an exploded star. I couldn't reconcile the image on the viewer with the living, breathing child next to me in her chair. Jasmine had enough brain function for essential bodily tasks—breathing, normal heart rate, and digestion—but she would never stand, never walk, never speak.

Yet Jasmine smiled and offered a rough sort of laugh at the sound of my "hello," when her mother wheeled her into the exam room. She beamed when her mother spoke to me of important events since their last visit. Jasmine had varying moods—some somber and withdrawn, others happy, even playful when I stooped to examine her. I have no way of knowing, of course, what Jasmine understood—in the way most people use the word—in these encounters. Perhaps she was reacting to familiar voices speaking in pleasing tones. Perhaps her smiles and laughs were no more than involuntary responses to sound, the reflexive release of neurotransmitters across what cerebral cortex she still had. If so, Jasmine's mother and I mistakenly read significance into her movements, sounds, and moods. But despite Jasmine's apparent lack of intentional action or symbolic communication, much less signs self-awareness, there was an interiority to her I recognized yet could not reach. Jasmine remained an unknowable Other.

What I did know—from experience and the opinions of trustworthy specialists—was that Jasmine had likely reached the peak of her intellectual powers. Decline and premature death would not be long in coming. I had no reason to believe Jasmine had any awareness of this. As far as I could tell, Jasmine knew no other time than now, no condition but the present. Her mother and I began an ongoing conversation about end of life care, including how aggressive she wanted us to be should Jasmine's breathing fail or her heart stop beating. Our discussions dwelt on matters Jasmine's mother would rather not imagine, but couldn't ignore. She consented to outpatient hospice care once she learned it wasn't an admission of utter hopelessness, that their services weren't leading the patient toward death but enhancing what remained of her life. I don't make many hospice referrals, and wondered which of her diagnoses qualified her for care, but hospice took care of that. Jasmine's initial assessment report listed her diagnosis as, "uncertainty of the future."

"Well, I have that, too," I thought, while conceding that Jasmine's case was rather more advanced.

Talking about things to come didn't distract us from business at hand: caring as best we could for Jasmine and keeping her as healthy as possible. In that,

Jasmine's mother was conspicuously diligent. Jasmine always arrived in the office clean, her hair done, her face shining, her diaper unsoiled. The useless muscles in her arms and legs were stiff and contracted, but not as bad as they would have been had her mother not been so faithful with her daily therapy. The white binder in which Jasmine's mother kept meticulous records of her medical visits and home care would make a certified accountant envious. No doubt all this attention prolonged Jasmine's life. At times, though, while I was writing my note after an office visit or leaving the hospital during one of her recurring admissions, I wondered to what end were we so industriously working. What was the point of Jasmine's life, much less that of devoting more time and scarce, expensive resources toward extending it? I'm old enough to know that a physician who denies having such thoughts is more saintly or less forthcoming than I. Questions of futility arise in the face of medicine's power over bodily decline. How does a community responsibly allocate scarce resources? What's the triage system for a needy planet? Does caring for Jasmine rob children on the Navajo Reservation or in Honduras? Is this a zero-sum game?

At least one reason, however, that my musings about futility remained unspoken is that I truly cared about Jasmine. Serving as Jasmine's pediatrician was more than a task. It was a privilege, a delight. Jasmine's mother cared, too—more deeply than I can imagine. She didn't idolize her daughter or make her the sole focus of her life as some parents of so-called special needs children do. She didn't blind herself to the consequences of the treatment choices she made for Jasmine. What she did so obviously and well was love her. Perhaps that was reason enough for me to keep at it.

But a parent's love for a child can't be the reason I care for many of my other patients. Robert, awaiting placement in a foster home, is as much my concern as Jasmine. So is Tyree, whose severe traumatic brain injury came at the hands of his crack-addicted mother's boyfriend. Tyree looks almost normal, if one ignores the appalling divot in his skull, but his limbs are already stiffening, his joints will soon twist at odd angles, and his boyish cuteness will rapidly fade. Few doctors get to choose their patients. In entering the next exam room, physicians tacitly consent to treat whoever waits there. If I were pediatrician only to the demonstrably loved, mine would be a very strange practice. What sort of love counts? How and to whom must it be displayed?

It wasn't simply Jasmine's approaching decline or present weakness that made me uneasy. Her disability vividly reminded me that my own status as a thinking, choosing individual is temporary and contingent. In the mean time—while I, at least, remained relatively able-bodied—there were no words to bridge the gulf between my professional and individual power and her utter dependence. She would never hike the desert with me, never share her thoughts and desires, never speak of things that make me come alive: books, music, art, and ideas. In all our time together, she remained a mysterious, unsettling Other. Mysterious, because what inner life she had was forever unavailable. Unsettling, because her otherness wordlessly shouted of the time when I will be as limited in my thoughts and choices as she is now. Jasmine, in reminding me of my body's inescapable contingency, was an affront to the life I live in my head. She frightened me with the silence of lifelong helplessness. In naming that fear, I recognized how much a misplaced desire for life without limits warped my vision.

As a pediatrician, I'm used to patients with whom I can't converse—infants both sick and well—but I find almost all babies cute. Jasmine possessed a certain cuteness, too, with brightly colored bows at the end of her braids to match her impeccable outfits. Infants, though, are often beautiful in immediately obvious and undeniable ways. It was harder for me to recognize Jasmine as beautiful, to look past what she can't do, to see the curve of her smile, the radiance of her eyes, the sheen of her mahogany skin. Nor was it easy or natural for me to stay in that posture of true sight, to keep my own body, mind, and heart in the present, to stop worrying about Jasmine's uncertain future. I wanted to see Jasmine the way Debbie effortlessly saw Roberto—as the most beautiful child in the world—but it doesn't come so easy for me. In a sense, Jasmine is an infant (from the Latin for "unable to speak"), but most infants I care for not only learn to speak, but grow into "productive members of society." Jasmine wouldn't. But in valuing my infant patients according to their adult potential to get and spend, I sacrificed Jasmine on the altar of commerce.

I like to think Jasmine was my friend, but it seemed easier for Jasmine to befriend me than vice versa. She smiled at the sound of my voice, not the clever things I had to say. Stripped of many conventional accoutrements of self, she wasn't distracted by those I'd spent a lifetime cultivating. She didn't appear put off by my temporary abilities and power as I was by her disability and weakness. She was an ideal Other, a perfect stranger, challenging me to overcome my fears, to engage her not simply as a partner in therapeutic alliance, but to welcome her in the practice of hospitality toward strangers. In time, I came to love Jasmine, but it took practice. I'm grateful for her patience, her long, silent waiting as I learned the necessary habits of love.

* * * *

Lauds ends as it began: in silence. A few monks remain in the stalls. Others attend to various tasks in the short time before the liturgy of the Mass. Two place candles alongside the altar. One sits at the small electronic keyboard, rehearsing a melody the monks will soon chant. Another ensures a wheelchair-bound priest has what he needs to follow along. His able-bodied colleagues emerge in liturgical vestments. No one speaks. No one hurries. Bells mark the canonical hours, the times when monks gather to pray, but there are no clocks on the wall to track the slow hemorrhage of the present: drip . . . drip . . . drip. In the embrace of silence, time moves from now to now in subtler ways. Through high windows, stars fade. Canyon cliffs take shape in early morning light. Red and buff sandstone emerges from black night, treeless layers of rock rippling toward a jagged summit. Above them, the first hint of cloudless day.

No doubt I should be preparing myself for Mass, too, but the morning sky is too beautiful to ignore. Until I lived in the high desert, I had no idea how much happened above me. Not that I appreciated what happened below. To me, plateaus, canyons, and vast horizons first appeared lifeless and desolate. I craved the sounds and diversions of electronic entertainment, the take home message, the useable answer. Small wonder deserts are called wastelands.

When white American settlers arrived in what is now called the Southwest, they complained native peoples weren't using the land properly. They soon remade the place in their own image, ultimately building cities like Phoenix and Las Vegas. They dammed the Colorado River to power air conditioners and water golf courses and front lawns. They covered square miles of red earth with concrete and tarmac that absorbs the sun's heat all day and slowly releases it into what once were cool desert nights. The Colorado no longer reaches the sea, dying instead in Mexican sands. Saguaro forests wither. Exotic plants choke the banks of natural waterways. Uranium tailings poison wells. In our rush to make the desert familiar and useful, we rendered our home unsustainable. We scarred the land.

Desert beauty is fraught, unsettling. It never hurries to reveal itself. Newcomers either accommodate to its pace or miss its gifts. Quiet helps. Silence frees me to see brown trout leaping at a cloud of flies, a four-foot long gopher snake taking the late March sun, a black-tailed jackrabbit shuddering beneath yucca spikes as a determined coyote paces nearby. Compared to the Eastern woodland habitats of my boyhood, webs of interdependence here are much clearer: sun and water, plant and animal, who eats what or whom, flourishing and death. Time slows, no longer measured in seconds on a wristwatch but in breaths, footsteps, and lifetimes. Simplicity sharpens the senses, purifies vocabulary, crushes sentimentality.

The Monastery of Christ in the Desert is a short drive from the late Georgia O'Keefe's studio at Ghost Ranch and her home in nearby Abiquiu. O'Keefe knew and loved this land long before I did. Cerro Pedernal, the flat-topped mountain about which O'Keefe claimed, "God told me if I painted it enough, I could have it,"[4] looms above Highway 84, just before the turn-off to the monastery. Her ashes are scattered on its summit. For fifty years, Benedictine monks have made their home not far from "her" mountain's base, thirteen rough miles of unpaved Forest Service road up canyon from the highway.

Northern New Mexico transformed the art of Georgia O'Keefe when she made her home here in 1940. Unadorned desert rewarded the practices of close observation she honed painting skyscrapers and flowers in New York. It was back East that she told a reporter in 1922, "It is only by selection, by elimination, and by emphasis that we get at the real meaning of things."[5] Her eye and heart found fertile ground in the desert, intuiting life in bare red hills, majesty in a bleached skull, and *eros* in twisting cottonwood limbs. Regarding some animal bones she brought back to her desert studio, she wrote:

> . . . they are as beautiful as anything I know. To me they are strangely more living than the animals walking around—hair and eyes and all with their tails twitching. The bones seem to cut sharply to the center of something that is keenly alive on the desert even tho' it is vast and empty and untouchable—and knows no kindness with all its beauty.[6]

O'Keefe's language reminds me of the way my Navajo friends talk of *hozho*, a word that rolls beauty, wholeness, harmony, and balance into a single immensity. *Hozho* has room for life and death, order and chaos, fine detail and vast emptiness. *Hozho* isn't pressed for time. A Navajo doesn't summon or control *hozho*, but walks in it. Words take on special significance in its silences. Reality conforms to language, not the other way around. Traditional Navajo choose words carefully, value reticence, sing often, and rarely shout. In this way, they resemble the monks at Christ in the Desert, who draw on a tradition that began when the first Christian monastics left the city

---

4. Quoted in Abrams, *Georgia O'Keeffe*, 97.
5. Quoted in *Birmingham Museum of Art: Guide to the Collection*, 144.
6. Quoted in Bry and Callaway, *Georgia O'Keefe*, 1.

for desert wastelands. Desert spiritual traditions converge on the need for silence and the power of words.

How foreign this is to the world of medicine, where beauty, like love, is at best a secondary concern and words are containers of information. Medical words are powerful not in themselves, but as tools: means to convey or enact desired changes. Traditional Navajo find Anglo doctors rude. Doctors, they say, ask too many questions. Navajo healers get to the heart of the matter with fewer words while most ceremonies last several nights. Anglo doctors always seem in a rush, eyeing the clock while they talk and talk and talk.

Yet my practice of asking many questions literally saves lives. There's a big payoff to the questions I ask and the answers I receive, duly recorded in the history and physical. All that talk informs my action. In the hospital, I have personnel and technology to enact what I say, and it's ultimately what I do for my patients that keeps them coming back. Doctors use words because they are useful.

From the viewpoint of scientific medicine, then, I've come to a very odd place: a desert monastery far from my machines, my team, and the trappings of power. I might explain my visit as a bit of R&R to boost my productivity upon my return to "the real world." Monks have no such excuse. Their work is irrelevant to the national economy. Their words make nothing happen. Their days are riddled with inefficiencies. The monks know they're very odd birds in a world of efficient power. I once heard Abbot Philip tell a group of visitors to the Monastery of Christ in the Desert, "We're useless. All we do is live here, work, and pray."

* * * *

While I served as Jasmine's primary care pediatrician, I saw her regularly and made frequent subspecialty referrals—neurology, otolaryngology, hospice, and so forth—as need arose. Jasmine's many consulting physicians seemed genuinely pleased to see her, but an outside observer might look at the time, technology, and expense and ask, "What's the use?" Jasmine's consulting physicians continued to see her for the same reason I did: Jasmine's mother brought her to us as a patient. Jasmine's mother makes medical decisions for her, as parents do for most of my pediatric patients, but Jasmine would never decide for herself. She had no words. She had no power or choice. She was utterly dependent.

Dependency and lack of choice are existential threats in a modern world though I, like most Americans, couch my fear in terms of utility. We want to be useful. "I don't want to be a burden," we say when faced with debilitating illness, imagining we haven't been burdens already and been so from birth. When had Jasmine not been a burden? In what years did her mother not change her diaper, not schedule her feedings, not drive her to her medical appointments? Much of Jasmine's brain was missing. Her arms and legs were withered and stiff. Grunts, smiles, and grimaces were the extent of her language. Few of us wish to live like that. Some think Jasmine shouldn't live like that either. In an ethical world that prizes lush valleys of possibility and choice, Jasmine was a desert.

I love deserts. I love their beauty. I love how desert simplicity trains my eyes to see the beauty in other landscapes. I love how desert silence teaches me to hear what matters. I've come to love Jasmine for the same reasons, though love wasn't my first response. It didn't come easy, but it's second nature to me now.

I love words, too, those deceptively simple works of art I wish Jasmine could share with me. I love the way words signify and sound. I love their ability to convey not only meaning but deep feeling. And I love words because of, not in spite of, their frailty. They never quite do what I want. Their limits and failures resemble mine. I would prefer them not to fail just now, as I try to put into words why Jasmine—who lacks so much that able-bodied individuals like me consider minimal conditions for meaningful life—should be loved. Words won't explain what I mean by her interior life. Words can't give a reason for her physician to love her. Words go only so far before they fail.

* * * *

It's Sunday at the Monastery of Christ in the Desert. Today's schedule differs from the rest of the week: all the canonical hours are there, but the pauses in between are roomier. It being the Christian Sabbath, there's no set time for work today. It's a day of rest. I speak with several of the brothers after morning Mass and catch up with Rosie, a woman who keeps a simple hermitage on the monastery grounds. She lives here year-round, another odd bird the monks welcome as a beloved Other. She helps them with outdoor projects and they, in turn, share their facilities with her where she leads meditation classes. I enjoy talking with Rosie. She's excited to tell me she's nearly completed her training to be a yoga instructor. We chat awhile before our voices trail away. Then we look at each other like two kids exhausted after a long, strenuous game, though we've done nothing more than stand and talk. We both smile, recognizing in the other a need for quiet. We say our farewells and go our separate ways. It's the most animated conversation I have all day.

After lunch, I walk along the dirt road that parallels the river. The day grows hot. I drink from my water bottle and wipe my mouth with the back of my hand when done. The brim of my hat shades my face and neck. I walk farther, turning off the road into a National Forest campground not yet open for the season. Empty campsites line the tree-covered riverbank. Under the shade of a cottonwood, I watch a scattering of insects flit over swirling water. It feels good to be out of the direct sun, and I linger awhile before moving on. Back on the Forest Service road, two younger monks pedal homeward on mountain bikes. We smile at each other. I walk in beauty and hold my tongue.

It's now late afternoon. We gather in the chapel for benediction and solemn vespers: a long period of silence we will conclude with songs and short prayers. I sit in a chair facing the altarpiece as the afternoon light slanting through the windows above us imperceptibly softens. I shift in my seat from time to time and hear other retreatants nearby do the same. Most of the monks have learned to stay still, while I'm like a hyperactive kindergartner. The front edge of the chair presses on my legs. Sweat from the hike clings to my shoulders and back. My body is here but my mind flits from place to place like a startled bird. Thoughts nervously alight and flap away, unbidden and unconnected. *What happened to the Navajo patient I referred to Phoenix for evaluation of a possible brain tumor? I hope she's back home and doing well. Have I budgeted enough time to drive from the monastery to the airport when I leave here in two days? What is the geologic name for the sandstone layer I see through the window? Does that monk always look that way or is he sick?*

Like a parent redirecting a curious toddler, I return my attention to now, here, and this, again and again. I'm not new to contemplative prayer, but I'll always be a beginner. Thinking, like knowing, is a strong suit for me. I think compulsively, if not always well. Introverts aren't all natural contemplatives. Quieting the mind is far harder than quieting the mouth. For all their years of practice, the monks still work at staying present. The monastic life isn't about fleeing the material world. It's a way of living into the messiness of dirt, water, bodies, and all the body takes and gives; to care for the things of creation without clinging. I look at the monks sitting in the choir stalls, some bolt upright, others leaning in their seats against the dark wood, their faces ranging from beatific to pained. Monks struggle, too, even in this beautiful place. I'm grateful for the company.

The words the monks bring to their "long loving look at the real" are very old: Hebrew psalms, first century Christian Scriptures, and Latin chants. The practice of silent contemplation is similarly ancient. It draws on a spiritual tradition known as apophatic (from the Greek *apo*, for "away from" or "other than" and *phanai*, "to speak") or the *via negativa* ("negative way"). Apophatic spirituality is inherently cautious, more confident in the human ability to say what God is *not* than what God is. Mystery is always more than we can say. Words, while necessary, take us only so far ("God is light") before they break down in negation ("God is darkness"), until the negation is itself negated in paradox ("God is bright darkness").

This isn't quite the same as the paradoxes of quantum mechanics, where the math leads to conclusions that defy visual models, everyday experience, and practical reason, but the resulting sense of bewilderment and awe is similar. Albert Einstein had considerable reservations about quantum theory, in part because of its indeterminacy, but also because it contradicted his understanding of physical reality. Einstein wanted theories to be correct and precise, but above all, he wanted them to be beautiful. I don't claim to understand quantum mechanics in anything more than a superficial sense, but I find its paradoxes beautiful. Paradoxes often are.

Einstein, whose religious thought tended toward pantheism, spoke confidently about the personal god he didn't believe in. The monks I know speak cautiously of the God to whom they devote their lives. Their language is planted thick with paradox: obedient freedom, God Incarnate, the Trinity. I try to get my head around the Christian doctrine of the Trinity—that the essence of the One God is participatory relationship—but my head is too small. Brother Christian, prior of the Monastery of Christ in the Desert says the Trinity is "so wonderful and sublime the human mind can't pretend to comprehend the full meaning of the mystery, but it's the cause of our joy and our hope." Joy and hope are visible in the faces of monks who live into paradox, who find beauty beyond words in unresolved tensions of mystery.

That beauty is best apprehended in a state of silent receptivity. There's a large crucifix on the adobe wall to the right as one faces the altar. It's covered in purple today for Lent, but I've watched monks and visitors gaze wordlessly at it in other seasons of the year. The crucifix is several feet high and done in the Spanish colonial manner common in Catholic churches of Northern New Mexico, the deeply moving folk art of a people more acquainted with grief and physical suffering than most modern Americans, including me. The image is deceptively simple and brutally unsentimental. The stylized body, or *corpus*, is stripped of everything but a pale turquoise breechcloth. The arms and legs are stretched taut, pinned to the cross by large nails. Muscles and ribs are visible under a canopy of skin streaked with rivulets of blood. The head is tilted, mouth and eyes wide with agony. As a central image in the church where the monks gather, the crucifix is a collision of opposites: life and death, chaos and order, omnipotent God and powerless victim. It's terrifying and, like O'Keefe's animal bones, strangely alive and breathtakingly beautiful; a wordless paradox where the essence of beauty is brokenness.

* * * *

Tim Lowly is an artist and musician living in Chicago with his wife, Sherrie, and their daughter, Temma. As a newborn, Temma had a cardiac arrest. Doctors and nurses restarted her heart, but lack of oxygen during her arrest irreversibly damaged her brain. I've never been Temma's doctor. I didn't work in that hospital or even in the same city, but I saw babies very much like her during my residency in Cleveland: infants in the neonatal intensive care unit, motionless from a barbiturate-induced coma meant to halt the storm of continuous seizures, slender clear plastic endotracheal tubes forcing air into tiny lungs, monitor wires and IV tubing snaking from pumps and machines, distraught parents at bedside, learning far too soon the impotence of parenthood, the inadequacy of words. I've also seen surprisingly healthy babies in follow-up clinic, weeks or months after harrowing experiences in neonatal intensive care. I've watched extremely small newborns flourish, sick lungs grow, injured kidneys recover, balky digestive tracts mature, and malformed hearts surgically fixed. Brains heal, too, but never so dramatically. While the newborn brain is resilient, its healing powers after severe injury are limited. It doesn't regrow. There is no mechanical replacement.

I first met Temma twenty years after her cardiac arrest. By then, she was much like Jasmine: medically complex, meticulously cared for, and conspicuously loved. My profession, however, habitually defines conditions and states by what a person lacks rather than what she is. Where others find presence, doctors see absence. In common medical parlance Temma is profoundly disabled. Like Jasmine, she rides in a custom-made wheelchair, will never walk or talk, and depends utterly on the care she receives from her parents and others. She's older than Jasmine and even more limited in her ability to change her environment or make known her will.

Yet a visit to the Lowlys is full of quiet joy. Tim greets me at the door, smiling broadly. He doesn't overwhelm guests with superficial talk. Our conversations quickly turn deep, intimate, revelatory. Sherrie is like a calm pond in a shady wood, beckoning visitors to stop and refresh themselves. Temma sits in her chair, the silent center around which the household slowly turns. I can't know how or if Temma marks the passage of time or what time could possibly mean in her experience. When I visit her house, however, time noticeably slows. The pauses between words grow rich with meaning. Space expands, as do moods and attitudes.

I came to know their family through Tim's paintings of Temma. For many years, Temma has served her father as model and muse. She is the subject of much of his work and an occasional model for his students. In the hands of a lesser artist or less reflective person, the relationship might have grown exploitive, but there's nothing of that in Tim's many paintings of his daughter. Realistically rendered in a variety of settings, Temma is broken and beautiful, damaged and dignified. She's revealed as what she's been all along: one of us, beckoning the viewer into the solidarity of self-recognition. She is also strangely Other, her painted presence silent and unknowable as she is in life. Temma is neither an object of pity nor the subject of spectacle, but a person whose outer form reveals mysterious interiority. Lowly's brushstrokes free me from the confines of professional jargon. His work introduces me to his daughter not through what she lacks but as the person she is.

Lowly's most haunting depiction of Temma is "Carry Me." Six women—Lowly's students—bear Temma in their arms. Temma's eyes are closed. She appears to be sleeping. Her clothed body is realistically depicted: her legs stiff, her fingers contorted, her proportions less than Greek. The other six look upward, directly at the viewer, with expressions of love and purpose. The tones are muted: brown and tan, hints of white and pink. Seven figures form an organic whole, Temma's six carriers returning the viewer's gaze, inviting us to share their common task without the comforts of voyeuristic distance. Temma is the center of a community lightly bearing her, neither an embarrassment to be hidden nor a problem to be solved. In ways my medical training can't articulate, Temma gathers those who hold her into a body. She isn't autonomous. She is literally a burden, however light, but her dependent presence—her body—transforms individuals into a people.

I gain much in seeing Temma neither as a wounded object of my professional beneficence nor the target of philanthropic concern for a few able-bodied selves, but as the unifying center around which a community forms. That insight, however, carries a high cost. It steals from me comforting assumptions hidden in the practice of medicine. Who really wields the instruments of healing: those who call themselves healers and helpers, or the one who calls them together? Where is the doctor without the patient, the healer without the sufferer? "Carry Me" deflates my illusions about who serves whom.

Equally powerful is an image called "Pillar." Dark at the periphery, the painting's luminous center is awash with red, gold, and blue blankets swaddling a sleeping Temma, her face and body turned to the side. Brown hair trails behind in the same direction as the partially turned blankets, as if blown by a wind or the result of a restless night. Temma's motionless body implies movement. She's a butterfly emerging from a chrysalis, her wings still crumpled, not yet ready for first flight. She is—like the painting—moving, delicate, beautiful.

Blankets cover much of her body, but this is clearly Temma in her broken beauty. Her hair comes to a peak on her sloping forehead. Her infirmities aren't painted away, but transfigured. In gold, red, and blue, the image resembles an Orthodox icon, a material window into a spiritual mystery. If the painting's title, "Pillar," suggests caryatids—carved female figures used as supporting columns in ancient Greek architecture—Temma's luminosity in the midst of darkness evokes a wilder possibility: the pillar of fire guiding the people of Israel in the Exodus from Egypt. She's a theophanous light in the desert, a startling presence, a disrupting vision. "Pillar" helps me see Temma as more than her physical and cognitive deficits. Though she remains a mysterious Other, my eyes apprehend at last that she is beautiful.

* * * *

I'm no longer Jasmine's doctor. I haven't been since I left my outpatient practice. I'm now an inpatient physician teaching residents and students at Cincinnati Children's Hospital Medical Center. My duties are full of new challenges, but I miss the company of families who called me their pediatrician. I still have the lifeblood of a physician's practice: direct patient contact and unmediated encounters with families in difficulty, but that comes in rushed hospital room discussions, not conversations taken up time and again over months or years. Sometimes I wonder if I made the wrong choice in leaving primary care.

I still see Jasmine when she visits the hospital. She's lived much longer than anyone expected, another reminder of the imprecision of medical knowledge. We last met by chance outside the hospital cafeteria. Her mother was wheeling her to a waiting van after an appointment with a pediatric subspecialist, and to my surprise and joy, Jasmine beamed at the sound my voice. Her mother and I asked one another, with genuine interest, how things were. We spent what little time we had together catching up. I had a strong and clear sense—immeasurable by any tool of medical science—of being in the presence of dear and knowing friends. It was good to be there, the three of us, together. It was a holy moment. "Holy" isn't the sort of language I use at hospital meetings, but it's precisely the right word, coming from an ancient root that birthed the words "whole," "heal," and "health." Meeting

Jasmine and her family in the hospital was a moment of wholeness, a healing encounter of souls. In a hallway outside the cafeteria of a major urban teaching hospital, I walked in *hozho*, if only for a moment. Our encounter reminded me to attend to the practice of presence in touching my patients, in hearing their stories, in sharing their grief and fear. On occasion, when I find myself perfunctorily examining the tenth child admitted this week to my service with an asthma exacerbation, or when I catch myself eyeing the door as a mother vents her anger and frustration at life in general and a dysfunctional medical system in particular, I remember Jasmine's smile, wordlessly calling me to be present. I don't know what lies behind her smile, what interior fullness it may betoken, but of this one thing I am certain: Jasmine's smile, like Jasmine herself, is beautiful.

* * * *

I'm walking back to the guesthouse from the chapel after Compline, the last of the canonical hours. The Great Silence, a time of special quiet lasting until the monks rise for Vigils, has begun. Pale moonlight falls on the canyon cliffs and crumbled talus slopes. As the desert's brokenness covers itself in shadow, I envy the monks who call this canyon home, who live every day in this holy corner of the material world, attending through its details to the hidden wholeness beyond. There will come a time when I'm too old and infirm to travel here. I will miss its harsh and simple beauty, but that time is not yet come. Grieving future losses is as pointless as wishing a better past. For now I'm content to be present, grateful to be here. It has been a long day rich with grace-filled, slow-moving time. I'm too tired to read when I enter my room. My mind's ready to obey the body. I lie on my bed, reflecting on the day, on Jasmine, on Temma. Then I close my eyes as the great silence settles around me like soft rain on waveless seas.

Chapter Fifteen

"Every Love Story is a Ghost Story"[1]

Cincinnati, Ohio/ Departamento de Intibucá, Honduras/Tuba City, Navajo Nation

AT THE EDGE OF an unvisited lawn of the University of Cincinnati medical campus, out of the swing of hospital traffic and hidden between the corner of a new parking garage and a row of liquid oxygen tanks, stands a lonely memorial. Midpoint on a small curving walkway leading nowhere, a bronze plaque mounted on a concrete plinth reads: "In Memoriam Cancer Patients/Radiation Effects Study 1960–1972." Below are two columns of unremarkable names and the phrase: "Presented by their families." The nearby bushes are closely trimmed and the surrounding beds carefully mulched, but I have yet to meet another person there. Perhaps the space was used for cigarette breaks before on-campus smoking was banned, but today no one goes there save the rare person who knows about the memorial and where it's kept. I've never found it on a campus map. When I first inquired, none of my colleagues had heard of it. If the hospital intended the plaque to rest in obscurity, few places are better suited.

Nothing on the plaque indicates those named were victims of experiments funded by the Department of Defense and conducted over twelve years by Eugene L. Saenger, a highly respected university radiation

1. See Max, *Every Love Story is a Ghost Story: A Life of David Foster Wallace.*

oncologist.[2] Most of the research subjects were working class or poor. Two-thirds were African-American. Nearly all were seriously ill with cancer when enrolled in the study. They didn't know they were receiving excessive doses of whole body radiation, nor were they informed of the dangers and likely effects of such exposure. At the time, it was believed full disclosure would skew the patients' subjective response data. Afterward, many relatives wondered why their loved ones died so quickly. It's difficult to know how many died from the effects of radiation exposure and how many from their cancer, but an outside physician who testified before Congress about the study called it "one of the worst things this Government has ever done to its citizens in secret."[3]

The doctors who carried out this and similar studies saw themselves—and were seen by colleagues at the time—as medical scientists and champions of progress. Dr. Saenger, who defended his research until his death at the age of ninety, never issued a formal apology to the families of his research subjects. He could never accept, much less reconcile himself to, the stories they told about him. He seemed to think his study patients were—or should have been—grateful for his attention and care. Dr. Saenger made significant scientific contributions both before and after the Radiation Effects Study. The American College of Radiology later awarded him a gold medal, and the University of Cincinnati named its radioisotope laboratory for him. Many colleagues were shocked at the criticism Dr. Saenger received after the secret study came to light in the early 1970s. They knew him as a brilliant scientist and consummate professional.

I never knew Dr. Saenger. I have no insight into his motives. I don't know whether he loved his patients or not. Perhaps he did—or thought he did—but chose a strange way to show it, though I suspect "love" wasn't an important consideration in his research design. As for his bedside manner, he likely adopted the professional stance of his mentors, who prized physician detachment. I'll never know what he was thinking as he irradiated people who looked, talked, and experienced life very differently than he did. It's hard enough for me to puzzle out my own motivations, much less someone else's. His patients are a cipher to me, too, though surely they came to the hospital seeking help, not harm. In the end, they had little reason to be grateful. For a brief time doctors and patients shared events that would, in the end, be life-changing, yet each person would, were they still alive, tell the story of those events quite differently. It was never Dr. Saenger's alone. The memorial is for the patients, not the doctor who deceived them. It's

2. Dicke, "Eugene Saenger, Controversial Doctor, Dies at 90."
3. Dr. David Egilman, Brown University, quoted in ibid.

important they be remembered, though I rarely walk there just to read the names of the dead. Mostly, I visit the memorial when I need to be alone. Solitude is guaranteed.

Well, not quite. Here, where I contemplate the harm even the best doctors cause, I'm once again in the company of masters and teachers no longer present—most of them patients, few of them white or well-known—from whom I learned the harsh and dreadful practice of a physician's love for patients. Harsh, because medicine's profoundest lessons are inextricably bound up with suffering and death. Dreadful, because it invites—and often demands—hard questions, regrets, and doubt. C. P. Snow remarked how "dreadfully vulnerable" we are through those we love. Any love, even a doctor's for his patients, requires a letting go, a surrender.

Medical stories are haunted by ghosts, bidden or unbidden. It's now years since Brian and Alice died. Had they had survived, I wouldn't recognize them today if we collided on a city sidewalk. Denied a chance to grow old, they briefly tutored me in their dying and seared images of their passing—Brian's enormous eyes, Alice's labored breath—in my faulty memory. They remind me how often medicine's reach exceeds its grasp. I couldn't control their diseases, couldn't stop their deaths, and they still trouble my most crafted memories like vandals toppling stones in a Zen garden.

* * * *

Months after caring for Jenrry and Roberto in rural Honduras, the two boys still haunted my thoughts. In one sense, we had saved their lives. They didn't die on our watch. Yet our farewells had been laced with uncertainty and dread. If "continuing in the hope" was a lesson turned necessary practice, it didn't curb my desire to know more of their story. I asked about Jenrry on my next medical trip to Honduras, hoping to revisit his weak smile, his grandmother's toothless grin, but without success. He and his family had vanished. Later, a clinic worker shared a second-hand story about Jenrry dying of what sounded like pneumonia a year after our brief time together at the clinic. She had no details, nothing to back it up. I never heard more. It's another story I have no control over, an uncertain denouement I'd creatively resolve were I writing fiction. I hope sometime to find what really happened, to learn how the story ended. Or continues. Until then, I still see him, smiling. I want him alive. I'll be saddened to learn that he's really dead, that I could live so comfortably, oblivious to his fate.

I had more success finding Roberto. Fourteen months after what I thought was our final goodbye, we met again. Maria, Roberto's mother, smiled broadly as Marvin, a Honduran doctor from the clinic, led me past the sloping *milpa* and into the family clearing. Maria was wearing—was it possible?—the clothes we'd left her in, the pink blouse open almost to mid chest, her long breasts barely hidden. She fetched Roberto and Santos from inside the hut—which looked a bit sturdier than before—and stripped them for weighing. Roberto had gained a few pounds in a year. Less than I'd hoped, nothing remarkable, but our fears of his imminent death proved unfounded. He seemed happier, delighted with the company, engaging everyone with his eyes. His heels were still tight. I moved them playfully, checking for range of movement. I showed some exercises Maria could do with him that might help.

Maria sat Roberto and Santos together on a slab bench by the back door and motioned us to take their photo. Both boys were naked save for pendants dangling from their necks on a long thread necklace. Each covered his genitals with his hands. I took one picture and suggested Maria put their clothes back on. The new baby was there, too—child number twelve by my count—and Maria held her in her arms. About a year old, she had an exuberance of black, curly hair. I snapped a family portrait. Maria's husband was nowhere to be found, but Marvin assured me he had been coming to the clinic every Friday to pick up food for the family. I asked Marvin about getting more calories into Roberto. "We'll have to see about that," he said, first in Spanish and again in English, though that phrase means the same thing in every language. I started to press him further, but he gave me a look I've seen before, the one that wordlessly protests, "You wouldn't understand how things work here." Marvin is a good man and a compassionate, tireless doctor, but he lived here full-time and dealt directly with the fractious *Comité de Salud* that oversees clinic resources. He had many patients with needs at least as pressing as Roberto's. I knew he wanted to do more for Roberto. More words from me wouldn't change a thing. I pressed my lips together, made a quick nod of my head, and began to gather my things. Marvin and I said goodbye and walked back down the slope to the truck.

Over the next two years, Jim and Debbie organized a support network for Roberto's family. Like me, they visited Roberto when they traveled to Honduras, but they were far more imaginative. Working with Rueben, another Honduran physician at the clinic in Santa Lucia, they donated money for targeted house improvements, including a water filter, sink, and latrine. Construction was supervised and installed by volunteers from Santa Lucia. When I returned to Honduras, I carried donations to Rueben for the next project: a concrete floor for the house to keep waste and parasites at bay.

My now fourteen-year-old son, Peter, accompanied me. He'd heard stories about Roberto and looked forward to meeting him.

Peter brought his video camera to Honduras to document our work. He has a keen visual sense. I've never heard a teenager appropriately use the word "beautiful" as often as Peter in Honduras. He inherited his father's love of stories and children. He especially enjoyed showing the Honduran children video of themselves. "A lot of these kids have never seen their own picture before, much less a video," he said after a field clinic. In the evenings, he kicked a soccer ball with the locals, handed out toys, or sat on the porch, taking pictures. His Spanish was minimal but language barriers quickly dissolved.

Through house calls and field clinics, Peter gained a sense of living conditions for the typical Honduran *campesino*. The morning we rode to Roberto's house in a pickup, Peter made sure to ride standing up in the back, where he could get the best view of the terrain. I sat in the cab with Rueben, who shared his concerns with me. The family had been doing reasonably well with their improved sanitation, and the newest children, born after Santos, were growing well. Roberto, however, hadn't maintained his weight from the last time I'd seen him. Rueben asked if there was something more we should be doing. He'd run out of ideas.

"Let's see what we find," I said, sounding more like Marvin than I intended.

Joining us on the visit was Marta, a physical therapist who had heard about Roberto and wanted to see him. Also along was James, one of the American doctors now staffing the clinic full time. James wanted me to examine a baby with cleft lip and palate whose house we'd visit on the way back. He narrated our tour on the road to Santa Rita, pointing out wildlife and telling stories about local goings-on. When we pulled over for the hike up to Roberto's house, we swung our packs down, checked our gear, and headed up the trail.

On our way through the *milpa,* James pointed to a hose running from our right—the direction of the stream—to the field. A weak trickle of water spilled into a full basin at the foot of a banana tree, irrigating it with overflow. No one waited at the hillcrest to greet us this time. We circled around the house and found Roberto's mother talking to an elderly neighbor. Maria wore a lace-fringed blue blouse open, as usual, nearly to her waist. Her latest child, a boy, was still nursing. I also noticed how Maria had pulled her green skirt over an expanded belly. Was she pregnant yet again?

We exchanged greetings. Children streamed outside at the sound of our voices. Santos saw we were gringos and started to cry. He wore a dirty T-shirt and no pants, but walked without assistance, hiding behind his mother wherever she moved. His wailing served as background for the rest of our visit.

Peter, who had brought a video camera, asked Maria if he could film as the doctors went about their business. Maria nodded, gesturing grandly at the house. I asked where Roberto was, and she pointed inside. Peter and I stepped through the door. Just inside was the hammock we'd given the family upon Roberto's return home, three years before. In it lay Roberto, the hammock's netted sides curving over him like a cocoon. He was silent, asleep, breathing slowly. There were small, healing sores on his exposed skin. A grimy white, pink, and blue baby blanket covered his groin. He'd grown visibly thinner, his right leg flexed toward me, the bony width of his knee contrasting sharply against the slenderness of his leg like a great knot in a taut rope. His hair and eyebrows gave him a feral look, but his sleeping face was at peace.

I gently moved his arms and legs to see how tight the muscles had grown. He started to whimper, and I half expected him to awaken and recognize me, but he kept to his fitful doze. Marta, the therapist, asked Maria to bring Roberto outside where we might see him more closely. We weighed him from a hanging scale we brought with us. He'd lost all the weight he'd gained after his stay in Santa Lucia. Peter watched silently, filming from time to time, clearly sobered by what he saw. We set a white plastic chair next to the table by the new water filter, and asked Maria to sit in it with Roberto in her lap. He was still struggling to sleep, annoyed at our attention. There was no engaging smile this time.

Marta bent to examine Roberto. "He'll eat better if you hold his head like this," Marta said to Roberto's mother, with Rueben interpreting for her. Maria smiled blankly and nodded. We'd been giving her advice from the moment we met her. Perhaps she feigned understanding just to make us shut up.

"He's so tight, so weak," Marta said with a grave look. "Does he ever leave the hammock?"

Roberto was weaker than I'd seen him before—not miserable like he'd been in clinic, but exhausted, drained. I wondered if his underlying developmental delay, the intellectual and physical limitations that prevented Roberto from elbowing his way to the table in the first place, were at catching up with him at last.

"If she's been feeding him all that she says," Rueben said, nodding in Maria's direction, "he should have gained more weight." He continued, "Either his underlying disease keeps him from growing or the food's going elsewhere."

When asked, Maria said Roberto was out of the hammock several times a day. She assured us he ate the beans and rice the clinic supplied. Rueben asked if she was pregnant, but she shook her head and laughed. She gave us all the answers we hoped for. Perhaps that's what she intended.

We weighed and measured the other children. Everyone but Santos was growing appropriately. I inspected the house. The walls were still sticks and mud, but there was an enlarged, if flimsy, tin roof extending over a small porch. I saw Don Roberto, Maria's husband, standing at the edge of the clearing, watching me with what looked like pride in his eyes and his bearing. How long had he been there? I greeted him and he nodded silently back. When I circled back around the house at the end of my visual survey, he was gone.

Before we left, I asked Rueben what the neighbors thought of all the attention lavished on this one family.

"Oh, they're okay with it," he said. "They know the family needs help. There were some people on the health committee who worried that Don Roberto drinks, but I told them we shouldn't hurt the kids because of what the father does. It's clear that some of the kids are being helped."

We said our goodbyes. I wondered once again if this was my last farewell to Roberto. Peter walked just ahead of me on the narrow path down, silently absorbing what he'd just witnessed. By the time we reached the parked truck, we were sweat-drenched and dispirited. James reminded me about the child with the cleft we planned to see on the way back. He knew the area where the family lived, but not the exact house. We drove half a mile to a shaded house with a large Pepsi sign in front. While James asked two local men if they knew where the family in question lived, Peter turned his video camera on an elderly man walking the dirt road alone, a satchel on his back. We followed the Pepsi sign indoors and bought something to drink, not knowing how long it might take James to find the right house. We were standing in the cool shade when James reappeared.

"Bad news," he said. "The baby with the cleft died last week. They already buried him. He'd been sick a few days and just died. The folks aren't around to answer more questions. Sorry to bring you out for this."

"Not at all," I said. "Sorry to hear about your patient."

As the truck reentered Santa Lucia, I noticed how much had changed since my first visit. Many streets were paved, the houses sturdier. Flowering bushes reached over well-built fences along the road. Whether because of the clinic or in spite of it, Santa Lucia looked healthy. For us, though, the day was a defeat: one child unexpectedly dead, another dwindling despite considerable effort. Back in the clinic, Peter slumped in a chair and looked over the film he'd taken.

"He's so small," he said, his words sounding more like a question than an observation. I wondered if I'd done right by Peter, bringing him to Honduras. Now he, too, knew firsthand that Roberto shared his world. He might have been happier or done just fine without knowing. I couldn't control what my son did with that knowledge. Not long after, however, Peter came home from high school with a challenge from one of his teachers, who asked the class, "If you say you care about the poor, what are their names?" Peter turned to me, nodded knowingly, and said, "Roberto."

The next year, a few days before Thanksgiving, Rueben emailed Jim and Debbie from Honduras with the news we'd long been expecting while hoping against: Roberto was dead. Jim called me the same night with the news. I knew from the sad, matter of fact tone of his voice what he had to say before he got to the matter at hand. There were even fewer details than in Jenrry's case: the circumstances unknown, cause of death unidentified. Like so much in his dozen years of life, his leaving it was mysterious. His family most likely buried him on the hilltop. Debbie recalls seeing at least one other grave marker outside the house on a prior visit, and was told another child had been buried there.

I thanked Jim for the call, said goodbye, hung up the phone, and went to tell Peter. My son took a long breath when I shared the news. His familiarity with death was limited—mostly to the recent passing of my elderly parents. Then he turned to me and said, "It was an honor to know him."

Then came the *coup* that exiled the sitting Honduran President in June, 2009. Focused as I was on patients over politics, it caught me by surprise, though there had been enough hints in the preceding months. Earlier that spring, I had returned to Honduras to help another pediatrician from Cincinnati Children's identify sites in Honduras where he might send residents interested in global health. We ended our search in the capital, Tegucigalpa. "Teguce" has never been a favorite of mine, but I tried to keep an open mind. During our hospital visits and meetings with medical educators and government officials, however, there was a sense that something important remained unsaid. We were received cordially, but no one was willing to commit. Seemingly offhand remarks about government uncertainty and "who knows who will be in charge" came and went. I assumed this was business as usual in a Central American capital. When we I flew home, most of our questions remained unanswered.

In late June, the Honduran Army, acting on orders from the country's Supreme Court, stormed the home of President Manuel Zelaya, arrested him, and put him on a plane to Costa Rica. This marked a crescendo in a festering political crisis, but not its end. Protests and political maneuvering continued, along with acts of violence and intimidation. Knowledgeable friends assured me that US citizens, especially outside the capital, were not in any danger. In the wake of the *coup*, however, government corruption and mismanagement, massive unemployment, and an exploding market for drug traffickers turned Honduras into the homicide capital of the world. As more sadness and violence unfolded, I felt a door was closing—for me if not for everyone. In time, Shoulder to Shoulder cautiously resumed sending medical brigades, but by then I was already headed in a different direction. I once said I loved Honduras and its people and I believe I still do, though others may tell that story differently. I haven't returned for medical work there in over six years. I know the door is still there, flush against the sill but unlocked. With resolve and effort, I could push it back open. Yet as the Honduran door swung shut, an old door reopened.

* * * *

I was on overnight call for pediatrics at the hospital in Tuba City when I received an urgent call from the Emergency Department. An ED nurse said a baby had arrived in continuous seizures and no one there had been able to start an IV, much less stop the child's convulsions. They needed me immediately. I hung up the phone and hurried over.

It was the middle of another two weeks of work in Tuba City, filling in as I did whenever needed. Much about the hospital had changed in the fifteen years since I'd lived on the Rez: facilities had improved, staff expanded, and serious acute illnesses gave way to chronic conditions like childhood obesity and Type II diabetes. The generation of children I'd cared for as a freshly-minted pediatrician were having babies of their own, inheritors of continued cultural erosion from the rip tides of historical trauma, poverty, and electronic entertainment. Children rarely arrived in the company of traditionally dressed grandparents, now being seen for their own medical problems by the geriatrician. Few families needed Navajo interpreters. Once, off-reservation boarding schools imposed the gift of progress on Native children, punishing them for speaking their people's tongue. Now, some children spoke little or no Navajo until they went to school, learning is as a second language. If a living language is the heart of a culture, the Navajo future may stand or fall on the how well this latest generation learns to speak *Diné bizaad*.

But much remained vibrant and familiar: Navajo reticence and readiness to laugh; humor dry as a desert mesa in the summer sun; beautiful lives; hard times. Doctors and nurses asked after Jill and the kids. Old work rhythms returned as I walked familiar hallways. Procedures I hadn't done in years and feared I'd forgotten how to do lingered in muscle memory. Years of difficult call nights, of having what residents call "a black cloud"—a pattern of horrendous medical encounters with the sickest of patients—proved the medical equivalent of battle hardening. It was good to be back.

I arrived in the Emergency Department and got the rest of the story from the Nurse Practitioner. A young couple brought in their three week-old baby who'd been acting strangely and was now making stiff repetitive movements. The ED triage nurse immediately brought the baby to a bed, where a doc tried to start an IV and give some medication to stop the baby's seizure. Three IV attempts had already failed. The baby was pale and unresponsive, her back stiffly arched, her arms and legs quivering. She looked dehydrated and headed for much worse. I couldn't find a vein worth trying. I knew what I needed to do: stop the seizure, obtain labs to figure out the baby's underlying problem, and replace lost fluids. I also knew I needed more assistance than the ED could offer, though the ED was far better supplied and staffed than it had been when I met Alice there on the night she died, years before. I asked the ED clerk to call another pediatrician for backup while I inserted a rectal tube through which I gave the baby some Valium.

The clerk's call was more successful than the tube. When Diana—Steve's wife and the most capable general pediatrician I've ever met—arrived, the baby's limbs still shook. I quickly recounted what little medical history I knew while Diana did her own rapid exam. We agreed the next step was an intraosseous (IO) line, a needle placed directly into one of the long bones of the baby's leg, the procedure Liz and I attempted without success on Jenrry in Honduras. There are now drills and sterile needle-drillbits made specifically for IO placement, devices that remove most of the guesswork and worry, but they hadn't yet made their way to Tuba City. We'd be going old school: twisting the needle into the bone by hand. It wasn't a difficult procedure, but the feel as the bone gives way to the metal tip unnerves me. Diana went to fetch needles, tubing, and other necessary equipment while I explained the plan to the nurse. I briefly considered letting Diana have first try, but decided against it. This was my patient.

In the end, my self-doubts proved unfounded. I slipped the IO needle into the baby's left tibia, just below the knee, delivered enough Valium to calm the seizures, and started fluids while Diana worked on stabilizing the needle with gauze and tape. We drew labs, ordered a head CT, discussed possible diagnoses—brain malformation, trauma, chemical imbalance, epilepsy—and where the baby should go once we had a handle on the diagnosis and plan. She was clearly too ill to stay in Tuba City, and likely needed intensive care in Phoenix. The diagnosis soon became clear: the CT was

normal, but the serum sodium, normally between 135 and 145 milliequiva-
lents per liter, was a shockingly low 117. Certainly low enough to provoke
seizures, but how had it gotten that way? A few questions to the young and
very frightened new parents solved that mystery, too. They had run out of
money for formula and had fed the baby nothing but water for more than
two days. There's little or no sodium in plain water, not nearly enough to
replace what's lost in urine, sweat, and stool. They'd meant no harm, but
their ill-informed attempt to help their newborn in difficult circumstances
had done just that.

In a surprisingly short time, we had assessed to the patient, arrived at
a diagnosis, started therapy, and arranged for transport to Phoenix. Diana
attended to the paperwork while I spent more time with the parents, reassuring them of the likelihood for full recovery, inquiring who would travel
with their baby to Phoenix, and otherwise directing their thoughts away
from guilt and self-accusation. They appeared calmer when they stepped
out of the crowded ED to call family and make travel plans. I turned back
to the exhausted patient, now sleeping to the up-tempo lullaby of the heart
monitor over her bed. Salt solution slowly dripped from the IV bag. The
IO line continued to work well. I asked the nurse to draw another blood
sample to see what our fluid therapy had accomplished so far. When very
low sodium levels cause seizures, the overall goal is to correct the sodium
slowly. Raising levels too quickly hurts the brain, too. By the time the flight-
suited transport team arrived, connected the baby to their own equipment
for flight, and began wheeling her to the waiting helicopter, the new sodium
level came back at 123. We were on track for a controlled recovery.

As we tidied up the messes we'd made in the ED, I was feeling rather
good about things. I asked Diana if there had been anything she would have
done differently. "No," she said, "You handled that well, though, if I were
you I probably wouldn't have kept my hand behind the kid's leg while I put
in the IO."

My eyes widened as I grasped what she was telling me. As I had pressed
the needle into the baby's small shin, I grabbed the back of the baby's left
leg in my hand for stability. I'd done no harm to me or the patient, but had
the needle slipped through or alongside the bone, as occasionally happens
when placing an IO line in very young infants, the needle tip could have
passed through the back of the leg and into my own hand. Not a fatal error,
but very bad form. It was a rookie mistake I warned interns against, the
medical equivalent of standing in the line of fire. In the adrenaline rush of
the moment, however, I'd ignored my own advice.

"No harm, no foul," I muttered, shrugging my shoulders, but I was
embarrassed. I took pride in my command of practices and procedures.

I preferred to point out my errors rather than have them called to my attention.

The next morning, as I walked to the hospital for another day's work, I crossed paths with Jane, another of the pediatricians who remembered me from the years Jill and I lived and worked in town. She knew my reputation for having brutal call nights with very ill patients and she'd apparently heard about the baby Diana and I had sent to Phoenix. She asked after a few details and I answered as best I could. We agreed the baby had needed quick treatment and transfer to intensive care. I made a point of saying how crucial Diana's help had been. Then Jane paused a moment, flashed a grin, and said, "Looks like you still are a shit magnet."

We both laughed at my reputation for bad luck on call. I recognized her comment for what it was: a battlefield compliment disguised as a barb, a comrade's acknowledgement of a hard job well done. A very ill baby came to the hospital. We did what was needed. She didn't die. Not this one, not this time. I'm grateful for moments like that, when I'm glad to be a pediatrician. In such moments on my return to the Navajo Nation, I was re-membered into the community. It felt like a homecoming.

On another morning, while working in the Tuba City pediatric clinic, I knocked on an exam room door, opened it, and stepped inside. The woman sitting in the chair along the wall turned from the toddler to face me and said "We're going to need some help." I shot a glance at the child, who was busily circumnavigating a chair, one hand holding on for support, the other groping for a plastic toy car several inches beyond his grasp. He didn't look ill. I wasn't sure precisely what the gray-haired woman meant by "needing help." I assumed she wasn't the boy's mother. She looked more like a grandmother, though she was dressed in a T-shirt and loose pants, not the traditional velveteen blouse and layered skirt.

I introduced myself in the Navajo way: a handshake with the lightest brush of fingers and palms, a softspoken "*Yá'át'ééh.*" She tipped her chin slightly downward and flashed the subtlest of smiles. I asked her why she'd brought the child in.

"He's got a cold, fever, and a rash."

"Just like everybody else," I thought, "and not very interesting." I was already rehearsing standard virus and cold care advice in my head while questioning her about symptoms, duration, and course. She seemed to understand what I was asking but had trouble answering clearly—more than the usual Navajo vagueness about time. I rephrased my questions, simplified my sentence structure. She looked at me with an expression I recognized as my own—that confluence of frustration and embarrassment when I had something to say in Honduras but couldn't recall the Spanish verb, much less in the past tense.

"Ah," I said, "You need an interpreter."

She smiled and nodded in agreement, generously overlooking that I needed an interpreter just as much as she. I excused myself a moment and stepped out of the room to the nurses' station.

"Haven't had to ask this in awhile," I said to the three women behind the desk, "but can one of you help me with some Navajo interpretation?"

One of the nurses followed me to the room. The three adults found seats as the child spun the wheels of his plastic car with his thumb. We would get to the history, exam, diagnosis, and treatment, but not just yet. I knew my interpreter would introduce herself in the Navajo way: her name, the clans she was born for and to, her immediate family and home. Then the grandmother would do the same. I'd have a minute or so just to listen, to prove than even a *bilagáana* can keep silent when necessary.

I sat on the exam table and listened to the slow rise and fall of Navajo vowels, glottal stops, and that blowing "l" sound over the tongue I'll never pronounce convincingly. My patient turned at the sound of his inheritance. He watched from the floor while two Navajo women breathed life into words I would never master. I smiled to think what mimics children are. If the culture is truly in the balance, scenes like this can tip the scale. *Diné Bizaad* wasn't dead. Not yet.

I found more projects that took me back to the Navajo Nation, pulling me closer to land and people with welcome bonds of affection and good work. Cincinnati Children's Hospital expressed interest in an Indian Health Service site where pediatric residents could work and learn. I made the necessary contacts and introductions, but another pediatrician and two unstoppable pediatric chief residents pulled the program together. My church developed a youth service trip to the Navajo Nation. We stayed on the grounds of the Catholic parish in Tuba City and spent the days working in the community, doing whatever people asked: painting walls and mending roofs, refitting neglected trailers, digging an outhouse in a Navajo sheep camp, and chopping fallen trees for winter firewood in a stand of pinyon pine.

Then came an opportunity I hadn't thought possible: one that combined medicine, writing, the Navajo people, and the desert. In the years I lived and worked full-time in Tuba City, several of my patients had inherited diseases unique to or unusually common to the western half of the Navajo reservation. Some had conditions we understood well enough to treat, such as Severe Combined Immune Deficiency (SCID), in which the body had no defense against infection without a bone marrow transplant.

Others had diseases we understood but couldn't fix—wasting diseases of the brain and liver. Still others had conditions for which we had neither name nor understanding. In the fifteen years since I'd left the reservation, much more had become known. Steve and Diana proved key in these discoveries, caring for the families while raising important questions for the subspecialists and researchers.

Among the puzzles Steve helped solve was the reason these conditions were predominantly found on the western part of the reservation, including a connection to the Navajo Long Walk of 1863–64, when Kit Carson, under orders from the US Army, forcibly moved Navajo people from their land to a camp in New Mexico the Navajo call *Hwéeldi*, "place of suffering." After four years of failed crops and dwindling numbers, the Navajo were able to negotiate a return to their homeland rather than further banishment to Indian Territory—present day Oklahoma. The US military mission was understood at the time as progressive, even humanitarian. That was the US Army's side of the story. No one asked the Navajo. That history is complex enough to merit an entire book, one that draws on cultural history, anthropology, history, medicine, and politics. To seriously engage this tragic history means asking the question, "When is a war finally over?" It's a story filled with ghosts.

The book took shape in my imagination, alternating modern-day stories in the voices and words of Navajo families, doctors, and researchers with relevant episodes in Navajo history. With permission from the Navajo Nation, I began tracking down and interviewing persons on and off the reservation. I knew some of the families from when we lived there. Others I met for the first time, with doctors and nurses serving as go-betweens, making sure families were open to talking to me. I drove highways and dirt roads, visited hospitals and hogans, and grew increasingly familiar with the Navajo landscape. The Navajo are often described as reserved, stoic, reluctant to speak of past evils, and all but silent about the dead. That was my experience at the hospital. Now, however, I discovered a readiness to share devastating stories and long-hidden tears. They honored me with alarming trust in my ability to tell their stories. The project acquired unanticipated moral seriousness: doing justice to narratives not my own. The book remains a work in progress, with many hours of interviews already recorded and transcribed, and much work still to be done. I intend to finish it, but I must do it well.

It was through book research that I reconnected with Kalene. When I lived and worked on the Navajo Nation, I helped provisionally diagnose Kalene's daughter—whom her family called "CP"—with SCID the day she was born. Kalene's family was well known to us: a previous child had died from overwhelming infection while waiting for a bone marrow transplant. During Kalene's pregnancy with CP, it was Jill who told her she was having twins. I was the pediatrician on service for the nursery when CP and her brother were born. After an exam, X ray, and a blood count, I knew the brother was fine. CP had evidence of SCID. I sent confirmatory tests while Diana readied the family for transfer to San Francisco for transplant. The transplant was a partial success: lifesaving, but with incomplete protection from the cells that make antibodies. Her course in and out of the hospital was complex. Diana was her primary doctor, but all the pediatricians came to know Kalene and CP well.

I lost contact with the family when we moved away, but Kalene remembered me. Once again, it helped immensely to be a doctor. While researching the book, I met Kalene and her family at the hospital, at their house, and out on the land. In the process, Kalene and I became friends. Our lives entwined in unexpected, sometimes painful, ways. She came to know my children, especially Maria. I met Kalene's extended family and grew to know CP as the funny, sometimes moody, and endlessly creative young woman she'd become. Kalene invited us to a family wedding. I shared her happiness when she found a new job and moved into a new home. I was in town when her husband and son were killed in a horrific collision on Main Street. I followed CP as her health declined, her lungs deteriorating in ways that baffled the doctors. CP's bone marrow transplant and subsequent medical care prolonged her life for more than twenty years, but not much more.

Just before CP died in a Tucson hospital, she told her sister, Bea, that she wasn't scared to die, but feared no one would remember when she was gone. "Oh, no," Bea said, "Everyone in your family will remember you. Besides, Dr. Brian is writing a book about you. You'll be more famous than the rest of us put together." Bea shared that story with me weeks afterward over dinner at the trading post in Cameron. She'd been fighting back tears as she spoke of CP's last days, but as she said the words, "Dr. Brian," she looked at me with sudden intensity and the faintest of smiles. It was the look of someone who, walking ahead, holds a door open, expecting you to follow.

"O, God," I thought to myself as I met Bea's gaze and received her story, "she's counting on me. CP's counting on me. This isn't just my story. Not anymore."

* * * *

I'm sharing a table in the dining room in the Cameron Trading Post with Kalene, Bea, and Bea's two sons. The waiter's taken our order. Kalene and

Bea will be having steak, CP's favorite entrée. The boys want burgers and fries. I've decided against the Navajo taco and ordered a large salad instead. While we wait for our food, Bea encourages the boys to draw with the crayons the waiter brought to the table. Her older son is more interested in playing Angry Birds on Bea's phone. I take a look around the dining room. The walls are covered with Navajo rugs and baskets. The ceiling is pressed tin. An enormous handmade pot stands by the stone fireplace. Tall windows overlook the Little Colorado River gorge, its sandy bottom dry until the next rain. The dining room is much larger than when I first visited the reservation, more than twenty years ago, but much remains familiar.

Kalene recalls my attention to the table, asking how Jill and the kids are doing. The two of us talk easily about family, jobs, and recent events on the Rez. We take turns dipping tortilla chips into a bowl of salsa, scattering tiny crumbs on the burgundy-colored tablecloth. Bea asks about the book, if I'm making progress.

"It's coming," I say with a wince. "A lot slower than I hoped, but it's coming."

"That's just like CP," Bea says, smiling. "She always did things on her own time."

I tell Kalene and Bea I hadn't planned on asking questions about CP today, that today was just a social call, dinner with good friends. "Maybe we can get through an entire meal without crying," I say, knowing that's unlikely. When we meet, it's usually Bea who cries, then Kalene. Sometimes it's me. It's a natural thing when talking about someone you love and miss and would do almost anything to see alive again.

The time for tears may come, but for now the boys are getting restless, unable to sit quietly in their chairs. I try to distract them with questions about school, but they won't be drawn in. The boys start to bicker over whose turn it is to use the cell phone and end up knocking a half-filled cup of water to the floor. Bea's sons remind me of Will and Peter when they were young, neither of whom could be hungry and patient at the same time. An older white couple at a nearby table turn our way and frown. "Tourists," I mutter, but stop short of meeting their disapproval with an icy stare. Maybe they've forgotten what it's like to entertain young children who are hungry.

And then, as if he'd waited for just this moment, the waiter begins sliding our plates in front of us. Bea helps the boys with the ketchup bottle. Kalene slices into her steak with a wood-handled knife. I lift a forkful from my plate. The dressing is sweeter than I remembered, but slivers of bitter radicchio lurk among the lettuce leaves. Quiet settles over the table as we eat. We'll talk again in a minute or so and someone will cry before we leave the table, but that's all to come. For now, I silently regard my companions, their lives and appearance so different from mine. I puzzle over the story I've stumbled into—too large to comprehend, too intricate to control. I wonder at the encounters that made us friends, the stories we've come to share, the loved ones we miss. I glance through the window at the red rock, lovely and fractured, the surrounding landscape unusually barren even for the desert. A hundred and fifty years ago, some of the Navajo fleeing Kit Carson came here to wait out the military roundup. What was it like for them, exiled to the edges of their traditional land, cut off from the familiar mesas and canyons their families called home? How could they walk in beauty while their relatives marched to a place of suffering? It astonishes me that the Navajo, after so much bitter history—including the Long Walk, off-reservation boarding schools, and a US government that harmed them more often than helped—aren't themselves bitter. Some are, but most range from resigned to determined to hopeful. Many are grateful to walk in their traditional land, between the four sacred mountains. How is that possible? I have so much to learn.

I'm learning to be grateful just to be in this good place with these good people, grateful for the many ways becoming a doctor led me here, grateful for the privilege of being a pediatrician. There are still times when I'm unhappy with my profession, but that's not now. I want to press into memory every detail of this moment: the eager faces of Bea's two sons, absorbed with dipping fries in ketchup; Kalene's soft voice as she tells me how CP made her laugh; the swirl of oil and vinegar at the edge of my dinner plate; the slow turning of the ceiling fan above our heads. I want to remember the sweet duty of delight whenever I'm reminded I'm not in control. I want to remember the gift it is to be grateful—here, now, and always.

Bibliography

Abrams, Dennis. *Georgia O'Keeffe: Artist*. New York: Infobase, 2009.

Augustine. *Confessions*. Edited by J. J. O'Donnell. http://www.stoa.org/hippo/noframe_entry.html.

Berry, Wendell. *Another Turn of the Crank*. Washington, DC: Counterpoint, 1995.

——. *Jayber Crow*. Washington, DC: Counterpoint, 2000.

——. *Standing by Words*. New York: North Point, 1983.

——. *That Distant Land: The Collected Stories*. Washington, DC: Shoemaker and Hoard, 2004.

Birmingham Museum of Art: Guide to the Collection. Birmingham, AL: Birmingham Museum of Art, 2010.

Bry, Doris, and Nicholas Callaway. *Georgia O'Keefe: In the West*. New York: Alfred A. Knopf, 1989.

Cairns, Scott. *Slow Pilgrim: The Collected Poems*. Brewster, MA: Paraclete, 2015.

Albert Camus. *The Fall*, Translated by Justin O'Brien. New York: Vintage, 1956.

Dicke, William. "Eugene Saenger, Controversial Doctor, Dies at 90." *New York Times*, October 11, 2007.

Dosteovsky, Fyodor. *The Brothers Karamazov*. Translated by Constance Garnett. New York: MacMillan, 1922.

Dunn, Stephen. *New and Selected Poems 1974–1994*. New York: W. W. Norton, 1994.

Forster, E. M. *Howard's End*. Cambridge: The Provost and Scholars of King's College, 1910.

John of the Cross. *The Poems of St. John of the Cross*. Translated by John Frederick Nims. Chicago: University of Chicago Press, 1979.

Max, D. T. *Every Love Story is a Ghost Story: A Life of David Foster Wallace*. New York: Penguin, 2013.

O'Brien, Tony. *Light in the Desert: Photographs from the Monastery of Christ in the Desert*. Santa Fe: Museum of New Mexico, 2011.

Osler, William. *Aequanimitas: With other addresses to medical students, nurses and practitioners of medicine*. Philadelphia: Blakiston, 1952.

Patrick, George Thomas White, and Frank Miller Chapman. *Introduction to Philosophy*. London: George Allen & Unwin, 1935.

Snow, C. P. *The Masters*. New York: Charles Scribner's Sons, 1951.

Solzhenitsyn, Alexsander. *The Gulag Archipelago*, volume 1. New York: Collins, 1974.

Steiner, George. *Tolstoy Or Dostoevsky: An Essay in the Old Criticism*. New Haven, CT: Yale University Press, 1996.

Thoreau, Henry David. *Henry David Thoreau*. New York; Library of America, 1985.

Traub, George W., ed. *An Ignatian Spirituality Reader*. Chicago: Loyola, 2008.

Volf, Miroslav. "Sarah Smith Memorial Conference 2008 Welcoming Remarks," http://faith.yale.edu/sites/default/files/sarah_smith_conf_welcome_2008_miroslav_volf.pdf

Weil, Simone. *Waiting for God*. Translated by Emma Craufurd. New York: Harper and Row, 1951.

Williams, William Carlos. *The Doctor Stories*. New York: New Directions, 1984.